Menopause the Way Nature Intended. Don't Sweat It!

KALYANI FAD

First published by Kalyani Fad 2021
kalyanifad.com

ISBN: 978-1-63752-372-8 (pbk)
ISBN: 978-1-63752-373-5 (ebk)

Editor: Consuelo Salazar

Typesetting and design by Publicious Book Publishing
Published in collaboration with Publicious Book Publishing
www.publicious.com.au

DISCLAIMER

This book is provided for general informational purposes and is not intended to nor does it dispense medical advice or other professional advice or prescribe the use of any technique as a form of diagnosis or treatment for any physical, emotional or medical condition. The author and the publisher assume no responsibility for the direct or indirect consequences of, and the reader should consult his or her medical, health or other professional before, using or following any of the practices, methods or suggestions in this book. The information provided in this book is not a substitute for medical or professional advice.

To my parents Luis and Sasa, no longer with us
To my husband Michael
To my children Juanita and Diego
To my eternal love, my granddaughters
Clementina, Yael, and Mattea

"If I could only leave one thing to future generations, it would be a culture of health. Being healthy allows them to reach their highest potential"

– Kalyani Fad

TABLE OF CONTENTS

Preface i

How to Read this Book iii

Chapter 1 Mindset for a Successful Midlife Transition 1

Chapter 2 Why I Wrote this Book 7

Chapter 3 Hormones for menopause. Are they the fountain of youth? 14

Chapter 4 Brief History and Scientific Studies on Hormone Replacement Therapy 21

Chapter 5 The Root cause of Menopause Symptoms. Actions Needed to Restore Health 29

Chapter 6 Healthy Pantry and Refrigerator. Reduce Exposure to Environmental Toxins in your Kitchen 42

Chapter 7 Mind/Body Lifestyle Practices to Bring Alignment to Your Life 54

Chapter 8 Rebuilding our Environment to Create Health 70

Chapter 9 How to Get the Best of the Food we Consume. Easy, Delicious, Nutritious

Sample Recipes 78

Conclusions 111

References 115

Preface

This book was written as a tribute to my mother and as a legacy to my daughters and granddaughters who motivated me to study and research this topic.

My passion for understanding the roles that food, nutrition, and lifestyle practices have in achieving and maintaining health has been part of my existence since I was very young. My decision to write this book and share my findings on natural solutions to achieve and maintain health came to me after learning how to obtain excellent health through my life by being conscientious about how I feed my body and my mind and how I have helped others to achieve similar results.

As a communicator, researcher (that like to question everything) and a holistic health coach with training in natural healing, I encountered the work of a former physician who uncovered an amazing truth: **Menopause is not a disease caused by hormone deficiency.** *In this book, I will reveal this finding, my own research, experience and the solution to eliminate* **the root cause** *of menopause symptoms like hot flashes, night sweats, weight gain… This is a non-invasive method without the use of hormones or drugs of any kind which totally eliminates the consequences of their side effects. This book shows you how to apply these concepts, using FOOD AS MEDICINE and how to*

i

incorporate mind/body lifestyle practices to maintain health and beauty during this period of life.

*My mother died of cancer and she also had a hysterectomy. My daughters and granddaughters one day will go through midlife change and I want to empower them with the knowledge and tools they need to implement a **Hormone-Free Solution for Menopause**, to help them have an easier midlife transition.*

This book can literally be a life saving instrument and can be the difference between maintaining vibrant health and vitality before (with prevention), during and after this period of life or having to go through the trouble most women experience because they think they have no more choices than following the conventional treatment offered by the medical system.

*This book is also for **you** and all the women in the world that do not want to use hormones for menopause and want to know a noninvasive way, a natural way to go through menopause and by doing so eliminating the exposure to the drugs' side effects.*

It is my intention that the information found in this book will help women to make an informed decision about whether or not to use hormones for menopause. I want to empower women by letting them know they have choices and they too can have the opportunity to live a fulfilling, healthy life to feel and look great by applying the principles given in this book: "Menopause the Way Nature Intended. Don't Sweat it!"

How to Read this Book

Menopause the Way Nature Intended Don't Sweat It!. is organized into 9 Chapters:

1. Mindset for a Successful Midlife Transition
2. Why I Wrote this Book
3. Hormones for Menopause. Are they the fountain of youth?
4. Brief history and Scientific Studies on HRT (Hormone replacement Therapy)
5. The Root Cause of Menopause Symptoms and Actions Needed to Restore Health
6. Healthy Pantry and Refrigerator and Reduce Exposure to Environmental Toxins in your Kitchen
7. Mind/body Lifestyle Practices to Bring Alignment to your Life
8. Rebuilding our Environment to Create Health
9. How to Get the Best out the Food we Consume. Easy, Delicious Nutritious Sample Recipes

In Chapter 1: Mindset for a Successful Midlife Transition
This chapter will tell you the rationale that inspired me to write the second edition. Why are we talking about mindset in this book? What is it that you can do to create the life you want at 50, 60, 70 and beyond? Discover it here.

In Chapter 2: Why I Wrote this Book
I reveal the real root cause of menopause symptoms and how by treating just the symptoms and not the root cause, and adding hormones to an already toxic body, make things worse.

In Chapter 3: Hormones for Menopause. Are they the fountain of youth?
If you are tempted to take hormones because you are been told they preserve youth and beauty, this chapter will show you what science has to say about hormone therapy and aging. You will be surprised. I provide a Natural and Effective solution to keep youth, beauty, and overall health.

Chapter 4: Brief History and Scientific Studies on Hormone Replacement Therapy
The main and largest scientific studies on HRT (Hormone Replacement Therapy) and their results. This information will help you to make an educated decision about using hormones or not for menopause.

Chapter 5: The Root Cause of Menopause Symptoms and Actions Needed to Restore Health
You will learn about the root cause of menopause symptoms, how the discovery took place, and the actions you need to take to restore health back into your life. I also cover other symptoms attributed to menopause and provide the solution. I will teach you a step by step method to detox the body and support the liver, and how to nourish your body to create the right environment for the body to thrive.

Chapter 6: Healthy Pantry and Refrigerator and Reduce Exposure to Environmental Toxins in your kitchen
I show you what foods to keep in your pantry and fridge to promote health, how to create a supportive environment in your kitchen, how to recognize toxic chemicals in your kitchen, and how to make healthy substitutions.

In Chapter 7: Mind/Body Lifestyle Practices to Bring Alignment to Your Life
Because of the mind/body connection, in order to achieve and maintain health, we need to take in account the person as a whole. I will talk about essential lifestyle practices to support the mind and the body such as: self-love and relationships, finding your passion and more.

Chapter 8: Rebuilding our Environment to Create Health
Recognizing xenotoxins (environmental toxins) in our homes: Our cleaning and personal care products, and other everyday items that are negatively affecting our health and what to do about them: Solutions

Chapter 9: How to Get the Best of the Food we Consume. Easy, Delicious, Nutritious Sample Recipes
I provide useful tips and recommendations to get *the best* out of the food we consume as well as some easy, nutritious, and delicious sample recipes.

I

Mindset for a Successful Midlife Transition

*"There are two ways to be happy: Change the
situation or Change your Mindset towards it"*
– Buddha.

First, let me clarify the rationality that inspires me to
write this second edition; and why the work in ourselves
and mindset is so crucial. We are experiencing a radical
change in the history of humanity that nobody was
foreseeing. This topic becomes very relevant at this time.
We are not going to ignore the socio-political realities
and changes we are experiencing. One thing I know is
that external circumstances can not define our future.
Society is always evolving as it did, for example, after
World War I, World War II, the Cold War, economic
depressions and recessions, and political/government
changes and upheavals, to name a few external
circumstances. And because of those changes, societies
evolve, adapt, and flourish.

I wanted to encourage women, who are the heart
and soul of the family, to envision and work for a better
world, and it all starts by changing the state of affairs,
which is where I think mindset changes everything.
Attitude changes our perception and the way we
experience life. We can see the world as gloomy and

hopeless and do nothing, or we can elevate ourselves to be the light to change what we can change. We should not let ourselves just blow in the wind.

Have you noticed that lately, in certain circles, everybody is talking about mindset? And did you know that this concept even existed at the time of Buddha in the year 623 BC! Why is it so essential to create the right mindset? BUT what is a mindset, anyway? And why are we talking about mindset in this book?

According to the Oxford English Dictionary, mindset is defined as a noun: The established set of attitudes by someone.

"Mind your life" What do I mean when I say:" Mind your life"? We can create life the way we want it and encompass what we care for in our life. Everything happens in the **mind first** - either as a conscious or unconscious thought- visualization or manifestation in our minds is the most crucial part of creating what we want. Once you have that clear vision in your **mind**, then develop an immediate, a short-term, and a long-term plan and make it happen by staying committed and focused on your vision and goals: **Mind your life!** Visualize in your mind the life you want to have.

So, since **everything starts in the mind**, this is what mindset is about: Like with everything that you want to accomplish in life, there are fundamentals:

1. **The most important one: You have to be clear about what you want.** You need to have a clear vision, goal, purpose of what you want to achieve.
2. **Preparation and practice.**

3. **Commitment and focus to accomplish your vision.** Remember, it's not about perfection; it is about commitment.

4. **And the most relevant, you have to have the conviction that you can accomplish your vision.**

Going back to the topic of this book, I'm going to share what my own experience, observations, and research have taught me about menopause:

1. It should not be a big deal to enter menopause if you are healthy, the periods stop, and life goes on as usual. But this is not the case for many women because they are not physically and psychologically prepared to make this process easy and they lack **the right mindset to embrace it.**

I will even argue that my program, suggested in this book, can also support women that have not hit menopause yet. Still, they need to start preparing their bodies and their mind before they even get to menopause, which is the ideal situation because prevention is better than having to cure. Postmenopausal women also benefit because they will maintain their health and vitality by using the tools I teach in this program.

No doubt that the knowledge you apply is power. This book provides you with a holistic understanding of what's going on in your body and how to stay physically and mentally healthy using the power of mindset, nutrition, and lifestyle practices.

2. Besides the lack of preparation, there are all kinds of myths and misinformation that women reaching

menopause have to face, like the cultural and social stigmas around this topic plus the financial motivations of the medical system trading on women's fears of menopause and aging.

In truth, what is happening is you are entering a stage of life that can be the most rewarding and exciting years of your life or the most miserable phase of experience, depending on your mindset because it's really up to you! It's all about your **Mindset.**

And let me explain! The symptoms associated with menopause are real for many women, which motivated me to write this book. Menopause - which is natural to all women, not a disease - has been medicalized and the "treatment" provided by the medical system is not designed to solve the real issue.

I am not denying the natural process of life: we all are born, mature and die, but no doubt, the way we think and what we do makes a big difference in the way we experience life regardless of the chronological age. The mindset with which we embrace life makes the difference.

So, what is the right mindset to conquer menopause? What is it that you can do to create the life you want while going through this process?

a. Have a **clear vision**, a goal of what you want your life to be, what do you want to achieve today, a week from now, a month from now, a year from now, in 5 years, at 60, 70, and beyond: How do you want to be, how do you want to look, what do you want to be doing, how functional you want to be, etc.

b. Design a plan to accomplish your vision, goal, and purpose. Monitor, observe results, and make adjustments to achieve your goal.
c. Start taking action NOW! You can not wait until you are 80 to say: "I want to live a long healthy life". You have to start NOW!

Committing to your goal or vision influences your choices and will become more intentional to accomplish your vision. For example, if your goal is to be functional, you have to involve yourself in doing physical activity: stretching, dancing, yoga, hiking, etc. Better than sitting on the couch and thinking you are old and defeated.

When some people hit the 50s or 60s, they think life is over because they have grandchildren, they sit-down and don't do anything. **Are you kidding me? Life is just beginning!** We have accumulated so much experience and we are wiser. It is the right time to pursue a dream or the passion we have postponed from the past. We can make a contribution to our families, communities, and the next generation by staying engaged and involved in the world.

Your food choices will also be intentional. You will start developing a healthy and robust connection with your body and engaging in activities that create stability in your life through daily self-care practices, etc. It could be that you don't know how to do this on your own, and you need guidance and this book will teach you.

Being conscious and committed to your vision requires effort and some sacrifice; and many people don't want to do this part because they don't understand that effort and sacrifice does not mean suffering. You will have to learn the art of "negotiation with your body" and present healthier alternatives that will contribute to your goal. Your body will be happy, and you will see the reward of making a healthier choice in the way you feel and look, and that is your motivation while getting closer to your goal. You have to enjoy the process; otherwise, you won't do it. This book provides you with the tools to make this "negotiation" easy and fun to help you reach your goal.

You will make the decisions in all areas of your life, such as relationships, social life, career, family, spirituality, values, etc., which will support your vision. You become the controller of your outcome. **Your mindset is: This is what I want, and I know I can make it happen!**

My contribution and my goal are to support women to learn how to naturally and effectively conquer menopause without the "aid" of drugs or hormones but instead using the power of mindset, nutrition, and lifestyle.

As mentioned before, women are at the core of the family. By providing them with the knowledge and tools to be healthy, we also help everyone in the family by creating a legacy of health. I strongly feel that if enough women join this movement, we will develop a healthy culture that benefits society entirely.

II

Why I wrote this book

Let me ask you this: what would it be worth to you to be able to go through menopause without experiencing symptoms and without using hormones or drugs of any kind?

If you are reading this book, you may be preparing to enter menopause or maybe you are already experiencing some of the following symptoms: hot flashes, night sweats, fogginess, fatigue, tiredness, weight gain, losing bone density, loss of libido, lack of sleep and more... and you are looking to regain health and confidence and don't want to use hormones but, you don't know what to do, which foods to eat to ease your symptoms? Then this is the book for you. The good news is there are natural solutions, non-invasive ways to bring health back to normal through natural food and lifestyle choices. This book will give you the guidelines to start implementing nutrition and lifestyle changes to retain health, vitality, appearance and magnetism.

The artificial junk "food" full of chemicals that people all over the world are consuming along with environmental toxins and lifestyle choices make people sick and age faster.

Modern medicine treats women's symptoms using invasive procedures such as screening and testing, hormone treatments and surgeries. I want to show women there is a different way, a natural way to address menopause symptoms. Through my experience, research and education, I discovered how to help women to have an easy transition to menopause using natural ways to achieve and maintain health before, during, and after their midlife transition so they have the possibility to have more energy, more confidence, and feel and look great which results in more productivity in their business or careers and relationships.

I personally went through menopause, some years ago, having no symptoms and without using hormones of any kind while some family members and friends, following the conventional treatment, have already had mastectomies, hysterectomies, etc. Women have been led to believe that many pathological states are normal just because they are common and this is the case of menopause symptoms and the way to fix this, according to modern medicine, is by adding hormones what worsen and masks the root cause. The truth is that normal menopause in a healthy woman is symptom-free, the monthly bleeding simply stops. *Menopause the Way Nature Intended. Don't Sweat It!* will assist you on the pathway to achieve the state of balance needed to experience optimal health and vitality during this wonderful period of your life.

Previous to doing what I do now, I obtained a degree in Communications and after finishing school I started my own cosmetics company which I successfully ran for fifteen years. But I have always been interested in the natural approach to health and I wanted to learn more about nutrition and health and all the different theories available. I became a certified holistic health coach. I also received training in Chinese medicine methods and later I studied with one of the foremost Alternative Healers alive.

I have always been a very curious woman. Since an early age, I found myself buying books about health and nutrition, the ones that provided information on prevention and healing using food and herbs as cures, not the conventional pill or surgery to "solve" everything. At that moment I was still working in my cosmetics business, nothing related directly to health. Later in life I had that aha moment when I finally decided to pay attention to what my intuition was trying to tell me for a long time: My path and passion is in the nutrition field to prevent and cure illnesses in a natural holistic way and maintaining health through lifestyle, food and herbs, as the famous Greek physician Hippocrates' (known as the father of modern medicine) famous quote: "LET YOUR FOOD BE YOUR MEDICINE AND YOUR MEDICINE BE YOUR FOOD". That concept is ingrained in my DNA and I'm really privileged to follow my passion and to share this knowledge with you.

Hippocrates' famous quote sums up an extraordinary truth, a phrase that, if it were taken into account in the contemporary world, it would help save humanity from disease. And since it was the father of medicine who promoted this, it makes sense that modern medicine should promote and practice this way of living!

Food changes everything; it becomes our blood, our cells, our organs, our thoughts, and our emotions. *The secret to prolonging youth and maintaining a healthy and vigorous life resides in the diligent care of the body.* The body is the vehicle that carries us through life and the way we take care of our bodies affects our life in all ways. As stated in the famous quote: "Healthy mind in healthy body", there is no doubt it refers to an intimate connection between mind/body; when you are taking care of your body your skin, your hair and your weight changes are noticeable but also your thinking becomes more clear, more focused and so influences your emotions as well; your life becomes more organized, more organic. This concept is very important if we realize our whole life depends on our state of health. Through this book, I will show you how you can experience an easy transition to menopause via knowledge, symptom-free through nutrition and healthy lifestyle choices.

Some women start developing symptoms of menopause in their late thirties but it's more common that symptoms appear between forty-five and fifty years of age. The mainstream belief is that the symptoms of menopause are a hormonal problem and a disease. That is what we were told by the doctors and the medical industry. Throughout my research and studying with a recognized former MD and Harvard Medical School Graduate Dr. Jennifer Daniels, considered one of the foremost Alternative Healing Physician alive today, I learned that it's a lot more to the story of hormones that what we really know and, how they got into the market. To learn more about this, since this topic is fully documented and I'm not going to re-invent the wheel, I recommend a book by Elizabeth Siegel Watkins "The Estrogen Elixir" Published by John Hopkins University Press, Watkins's book goes into depth and detail, accurately and impartiality on the evolution of

10

menopausal hormone therapy and its promises to women to prolong youth and prevent the diseases of aging. The truth is that hormones are neither the answer nor the fountain of youth. They are going to give patients a lot of unnecessary pain and suffering because of the side effects that will interfere with their quality of life.

Of course, it's a personal decision whether to use hormones for menopause or not but, this decision should be an educated decision.

My intention with this book is to make women realize that they do have choices in how they approach menopause and providing the information to allow them to decide which direction they want to choose. If they choose the hormone free solution for menopause, the tools in this book helps them have an easier midlife transition through the use of natural foods, nutrition, and lifestyle practices.

What is menopause? It's the stop of menstrual cycles for one full year. The symptoms of female midlife linked to the ending of periods and called menopause is now accepted to be a disease caused by the decrease of hormones and mainstream medicine treats the symptoms by prescribing hormones, artificial or bio-identicals.

But is it really a condition caused by hormones?

According to conventional medicine, all of these symptoms associated with the absence of periods are supposedly caused by the lack of hormones, and then hormones are prescribed to treat the **symptoms**, but not the root cause.

Studying with Dr. Daniels I learned **that the root cause** is the toxins accumulated in the blood when women stop menstruation and the toxins aren't flowing out with the monthly bleeding. For instance, hot flashes have nothing to do with hormones, it's the unexpected concentration of toxins and chemicals in the blood and the body is not prepared for this extreme level of toxins. The body then creates a big heat, pushes out to the skin and disposes of the toxins by perspiration which we call hot flashes.

When you take hormones that stop the hot flashes, the toxins accumulate and that is how you get the increase of heart attacks, increase of stroke and an array of other problems because what you have done is preventing the disposal of these toxins through the right channels and they begin to accumulate even more.

So the way to get rid of menopause symptoms is to provide the toxins (the root cause) another way out of the body and in this book will show you how to do it.

The hormone-free solution for menopause helps you retain...helps you to retain your youthful look, vitality, and confidence. By using diet, nutrition and lifestyle practices, you will learn how to eliminate the uncomfortable symptoms of peri-menopause or menopause and completely eradicate the risk of the side effects related to hormone replacement therapy (HRT)[1] either, (HRT) FDA[2] approved[3] or the so-called Bio-identicals[4] such as cancer, heart disease, stroke, blood clots in the lung, increased risk of dementia and more[5].

---

1. HRT stands for "hormone replacement therapy"
2. Food and Drug Administration
3. https://www.menopause.org/publications/clinical-practice-materials/government-approved-drugs-for-menopause
4. https://www.health.harvard.edu/womens-health/bioidentical-hormones-help-or-hype
https://www.fda.gov/ForConsumers/ConsumerUpdates/ucm107836.htm
http://www.pharmwatch.org/strategy/bioidentical.shtml
5. https://www.nlm.nih.gov/databases/alerts/estrogen_progestin.html

Taking hormones is not the solution to ease menopause symptoms. Menopause is not a disease caused by decline of hormones, it's a natural phase in women's lives and the hormone-free solution for menopause will assist you through this transition using a natural, holistic method that supports elimination of toxins through the right channels as well as providing the proper nutrition and lifestyle choices to reach homeostasis to regain health and well being. The only side effects you might experience with the hormone-free solution for menopause is that you also recover from other illnesses you may have since we treat the whole person not just the symptoms.

By implementing the nutritional and lifestyle recommendations given here you start experiencing noticeable improvements of all your symptoms.

You will learn: the amount and type of water to drink, how to clean up your diet, how to aid with the elimination process through the right channels, how to stock a healthy pantry and fridge and essential lifestyle mind/ body practices, as well as how to recognize and get rid of environmental toxins that are destroying your health.

|||

Hormones for menopause.
Are they the fountain of youth?

"Beauty is mostly an inner job"
– Kalyani Fad

Why am I adding this chapter in this new edition? One common trend I have noticed is that some women are "tempted" to take hormones just because they have been sold the idea that taking hormones for menopause is the way to preserve youth and beauty.[1] I want to develop this topic because after all, who doesn't want to be forever young? But, of course, you don't want to die in the attempt! My goal is to provide clarity in the storm of misinformation.

Based on my experience, observation and extensive research, it is evident to me that when women follow the trend of taking dangerous chemicals (hormones) for menopause as the fountain of youth they don't only not look or feel young but, instead, they are exposing themselves to the risk – as demonstrated in the largest scientific studies[2] of the harmful side effects of hormone therapy like cancers, heart disease, strokes, dementia and

1. https://jamanetwork.com/journals/jama/article-abstract/660431
2. https://wayback.archive-it.org/org-350/20200921200315/https://www.nlm.nih.gov/databases/alerts/estrogen_progestin.html

more. And, as we all know, it's very difficult to exude youth, vibrancy and happiness when we are sick.

Let me explain my position about this topic **taking into account what Science has to say about aging and hormone therapy of any kind.** I came across a paper published by The National Institute on Aging (NIA), part of the Federal Government's National Institutes of Health (NIH) called: "Can We Prevent Aging?" [3] According to this paper adding external hormones to keep beautiful skin and hair or to stop the aging process not only does not work but instead causes harmful side effects because, among others, adding external hormones disturbs the natural balance of hormones in the body.

"Because hormonal balance is so intricate, too much of a hormone in your system may actually cause the opposite of the intended effect. For example, taking a hormone supplement can cause your own hormone regulation to stop working. Or, your body may process the supplements differently than the naturally produced hormone, causing an alternate, undesired effect. It is also possible that a supplement could amplify negative side effects of the hormone naturally produced by the body. At this point, scientists do not know all the consequences."

The paper also points out the marketing strategy to keep consumers for life using fear and false promises:

"You may have read magazine articles or seen television programs suggesting that treatment with hormones can make people feel young again or can slow or prevent aging. That's because finding a "fountain of youth" is a captivating story.

---

3. http://www.isoad.org/Assets/userfiles/sys_eb538c1c-65ff-4e82-8e6a-a1ef01127fed/fi les/Resouce/can_we_prevent_aging_0.pdf

The truth is that, to date, no research has shown that hormone therapies add years to life or prevent age-related frailty."

Yes, your hormones decline during our lifetime by nature's design – but you don't try to correct nature. When you take hormones for menopause you are playing with fire as study after study has shown.[4]

"Higher concentrations of hormones in your body are not necessarily better. And, a decrease in hormone concentration with age is not necessarily a bad thing. The body maintains a delicate balance between how much hormone it produces and how much it needs to function properly. Natural hormone production fluctuates throughout the day. That means that the amount of hormone in your blood when you wake up may be different 2, 12, or 20 hours later".

The research notes, what we already have known for a long time: "there is positive evidence for the health benefits of adding whole fruits and vegetables to the diet" and concludes that "It is important to remember there is already plenty of research supporting the value of a healthy, balanced diet and physical activity to help delay or prevent age-related problems."

Maintaining a healthy diet is the way to go to maintain youth and beauty: *"Fruit and vegetables consumption may represent the most healthy and safe method in order to maintain a balanced diet and youthful appearing skin."* [5]

---

4. https://wayback.archive-it.org/org-350/20200921200315/https://www.nlm.nih.gov/databases/alerts/estrogen_progestin.html
5. https://www.ncbi.nlm.nih.gov/pmc/articles/PMC3583891/

What is the secret to extending youth?

This is what I have learned through the years, natural wholesome foods and lifestyle choices along with a healthy mind and mindset are the key to vibrant health that will reflect in your skin, hair and your overall appearance.

One thing is for sure: Hormones DON'T MAKE YOU BEAUTIFUL OR AGELESS, instead they get you in trouble and they are not good for you as explained above. You can read it here in this book, or do your own research about the harmful side effects of hormone therapy.

The diet promotes health and definitely will show up in the condition of your skin and hair, nails, etc. I recommend consuming organic wholesome fruits and vegetables, whole grains, collagen promoting foods and healthy fats. Wrinkled dried skin is caused by malnutrition. Lack of collagen is one of the deficiencies.[6] Also, avoid junk processed foods that are full of rancid oils and chemicals which generate toxins and cause malnutrition because they have nutrients scarcity.

A youthful and healthy appearance is a combination of actions; no magic cream or drug can do that for you. I have seen women that have never used hormones for menopause, who are health conscious and they have beautiful skin and hair. I personally stay away from hormones and I get a lot of compliments about my hair and my skin.

A healthy person is an attractive person showing in his/her attitude towards life and even in her/his posture. You can do a lot to prolong the youthful appearance regardless

---

6. https://www.ncbi.nlm.nih.gov/pmc/articles/PMC3583891/

of your chronological age easily. It all goes back to your thoughts, mindset, how do you want to feel, look, and what you do at every stage of your life. You need a clear vision, plans, and strategies to execute your vision.

So, there is an internal practice to do that involves the way we feed our body and also our mind. The body's work requires diet, hydration, cleansing, etc. as explained in this book.

But, it's deeper than that, not all the work is physical because of the mind/body connection, your body feels everything your mind creates, "positive" or "negative ", we are psychosomatic. We have to take in account our thoughts, the way we perceive life, our state of mind. It is crucial to have a positive approach to life and a purpose in life, something to look forward to and that motivates you, something that "makes your heart sing" to maintain health, beauty and youthful appearance. Whatever that is for you, I call this enthusiasm to live.

Unresolved emotions and conflicts: anger, fear, anxiety, regrets, envy, resentment, dissatisfaction, worry, sorrow, etc. show up in your face's expressions because you are tensing certain facial muscles that create wrinkles not to mention the negative impact those kind of emotions have on your overall health, (they poison you, not other people you have the conflict with) causing cancer,[7] cardiovascular events,[8] diabetes,[9] among others.

Of course, some of the wrinkles are the result of a lot of laughter. And, I'm okay with those! *"Laughter is the best*

7. https://www.cancerwisdom.net/stress-and-cancer/
8. https://academic.oup.com/eurheartj/article/35/21/1404/583173
9. https://www.ncbi.nlm.nih.gov/pmc/articles/PMC3019061/

Medicine" this quote is attributed to Henri de Mondeville a professor of surgery who lived in the 1300s and propagated post-operative therapy with humor.

Chronic stress, caused by an ongoing unsolved situation or the sense of un-fulfillment, is a good recipe for aging. Aside from the effects that a worried face has on facial wrinkles, stress affects your health by suppressing the immune system, causing all kind of illnesses that speeds up the aging process and actually can end up killing you. So, you really have to work in the issues that are causing you that kind of stress, do what it takes to remove yourself from that situation.

I do focus on all the above factors, because we really glow and radiate beauty from the inside. Also, I **do** stay away from commercial creams, and synthetic beauty products, soaps, and perfumes, that basically destroys the skin and contribute to the toxicity in the body because your body absorbs these chemicals.

My perspective about skin care and about everything else for that matter, is to work in harmony with nature. I avoid invasive or harsh man-made chemicals in my body and in my environment.

I feed my skin from the outside by using 100% organic, cold pressed oils because they help maintain the moisture and integrity of the outer layer of the skin. I use them for cleansing, exfoliating, and as a moisturizer.

1. To cleanse and exfoliate, use a carrier oil like jojoba, castor, olive etc. combined with a few drops of essential oils like frankincense or sandalwood. You can use any combination you like. My favorite is rosehip oil because it's rich in vitamin C[10] which

10. https://www.ncbi.nlm.nih.gov/pmc/articles/PMC3673383/

stimulates collagen production, and it also combats wrinkles. Apply a few drops on the skin, massage upwards in a circular motion.

2. Damp a cotton washcloth in warm water, apply it on the face and press to make a steam to activate the oils and wipe. Or just damp a small portion of a cotton washcloth and put a few drops of your favorite oil, massage gently to cleanse or energetically to exfoliate the skin.

3. Add moisture if you desire by applying a few drops of your favorite combination of oils, I combine a carrier oil like rosehip, olive, castor, coconut, almond, jojoba oil with 2 or 3 drops of essential oils of your preference like turmeric, myrrh, ylang, and carrot seed which are excellent to keep the skin's elasticity. I also like frankincense for fine lines.

And finally and very importantly: do not get into the trap limitations and programing about your chronological age, *just enjoy your life* without the culturally and socially imposed restrictions or your own self-imposed limitations about age that dictates how you should look, what you should do or or not do because of your chronological age. *Don't think about age, don't talk about age!* ***Please don't do it, it is very liberating!***

My conclusion: Beauty and youth are mostly an internal work – what eat and what we think - and where we should concentrate most of our effort. **Mind your Life!**

IV

Brief History and Scientific Studies on Hormone Replacement Therapy

Talking with many of my clients, I have noticed there is an increase of diseases, especially in cancer and other ailments in women taking HRT (Hormone Replacement Therapy) as a way to alleviate their menopause symptoms.

All drugs have adverse side effects and HRT (Hormone replacement therapy) is not the exception. Women, in general, don't know much about them and doctors don't talk too much about them either. They are just overlooked[6].

For this reason, I decided to write this chapter in case you are interested in knowing what are the findings and results of some of the biggest and most important scientific studies on the topic of Hormone Replacement Therapy. It's my hope that women will find this informative and will help them make an educated decision about whether or not HRT is what they want to do.

---

6. https://www.ncbi.nlm.nih.gov/pmc/articles/PMC2935455/

Brief History of HRT and Main Scientific Studies

–   The pharmaceutical development of estrogen therapy began in the 1930's in the USA but really took off in the years after World War II. This was the beginning of the commercialization of estrogen.

–   Since the early beginnings of estrogen therapy, the collaborators in the isolation of estrogen in the US **identified and warned about the cancer link associated with adding estrogen** in a 1940 article published in The Journal of American Medical Association (JAMA)[7].

–   In 1942 the FDA approved a drug called Premarin (estrogen from pregnant mares' urine) for the treatment of menopausal symptoms and the drug was looking for a market[8].

Initially, Premarin didn't get too much acceptance and found a lot of resistance from doctors and women. From 1930 to 1950, based on the cautionary articles in medical journals like the editorial called "Estrogen Therapy-A Warning" published in The Journal of the American Medical Association JAMA in December 1939 and many others published on both continents, doctors only

7. http://jamanetwork.com/journals/jama/article-abstract/1160379?resultClick=1
8. https://www.ncbi.nlm.nih.gov/pubmed/23974785

used estrogens in very few extreme cases and instead advised women to have a balanced diet, avoidance of stress and sometimes prescribed sedatives as a more conservative way to treat the symptoms of menopause[9].

– In the late 1960's, they were prescribed and promoted as a wonder drug benefiting health, vitality, and femininity and also to stop the aging process. The book "Feminine Forever" by physician Robert Wilson in 1966 was a great contributor to this hype, claiming that HRT's miraculous effects in restoring women's youth, beauty, and sexuality.[10]

– Doctors started prescribing Hormone replacement therapy (HRT) and women started using HRT until studies showed that estrogens increase endometrial cancer. In 1975 studies showed how endometrial cancer cases had risen in the mid-1960's and reached a peak in 1975 caused by estrogen replacement therapy. They discovered over 15,000 cases from 1971-1975 in the western United States where estrogen replacement therapy was used.

"This represents one of the largest epidemics of serious iatrogenic disease that has ever occurred in the country. With the substantial fall in estrogen sales in January 1976, there has been

9. From the book: "The Estrogen Elixir" pages 33, 34
10. http://jamanetwork.com/journals/jama/article-abstract/660431

an associated decline in the incident rates of endometrial cancer nationwide."[11]

Sales of Hormone Replacement Therapy (HRT) started to drop but a decade later these studies were already forgotten and HRT sales began to increase again especially because pharmaceutical companies came up with another drug called Prempro, a combination of estrogen and progestin to supposedly avoid endometrial cancer, but Prempro also showed to create more invasive breast cancers, heart attacks, strokes, blood clots… I'm quoting an article dated September 2005 in the US National Library of Medicine:

"asking why, for four decades, since the mid-1960s, were millions of women prescribed powerful pharmacological agents already demonstrated, three decades earlier, to be carcinogenic? Answering this question requires engaging with core issues of accountability, complexity, fear of mortality, and the conduct of socially responsible science[12].*"*

Premarin continued being promoted to prevent especially osteoporosis and heart disease and in 1992 it became the most frequently prescribed drug in the US for the rest of the century.[13]

11. http://ajph.aphapublications.org/doi/abs/10.2105/AJPH.70.3.264
12. https://www.ncbi.nlm.nih.gov/pmc/articles/PMC1733142
13. https://books.google.com/books?id=EFI7tr9XK6EC&pg=RA1-PA481&lpg=RA1-PA481&dq=%22Premarin++to+prevent+osteoporosis+and+heart+disease+and+in+1992+it+became+the+most+frequently+prescribed+drug+in+the+US+for+the+rest+of+the+century&source=bl&ots=o_bSV-dAfI&sig=wVBmKyBIasqBK2PUPrjXU3eimLo&hl=en&sa=X&ved=0ahUKEwjD0o-a_9DWAhWJsFQKHQNiBa8Q6AEIKDAA#v=onepage&q&f=false
https://books.google.com/books?id=a15VI2I-4NgC&pg=PT53&lpg=PT53&dq=Premarin++to+prevent+osteoporosis+the+most+prescribed+drug+for+the+rest+of+the+century&source=bl&ots=q-6IlV-p3D&sig=aQJhAS22I_sR9jLOMYp73RZL7ec&hl=en&sa=X&ved=0ahUKEwj6p76vgtHWAhVM0FQKHaR0DkkQ6AEIKjAA#v=onepa

– In 2002 a huge federal study on hormone therapy called **The Women's Health Initiative (WHI)** was terminated three years before completion because "the harm was greater than the benefit" after researchers found that participants that took the combined estrogen and progestin had an increased invasive breast cancer, heart disease, strokes, and pulmonary embolisms compared to women taking placebo pills. A later study also showed increase of dementia in older patients.

"Specific study findings for the estrogen plus progestin group compared to placebo include:

- A 41 percent increase in strokes
- A 29 percent increase in heart attacks
- A doubling of rates of venous thromboembolism (blood clots)
- A 22 percent increase in total cardiovascular disease
- A 26 percent increase in breast cancer[14]."

After such devastating results, some women changed to bioidenticals, believing that they were superior as they were promoted by celebrities as role models. The story is repeating again but this time with the bioidentical hormones which are also synthetic because to make products that work for humans, raw materials from plants have to be converted to human hormones

ge&q=Premarin to prevent osteoporosis the most prescribed drug for the rest of the century&f=false

14. https://www.nhlbi.nih.gov/news/press-releases/2002/nhlbi-stops-trial-of-estrogen-plus-progestin-due-to-increased-breast-cancer-risk-lack-of-overall-benefit

synthetically[15]. Neither the synthetic ones nor the so-called bioidenticals are safe because they both are external hormones and we already know what added hormones for menopause cause.

The symptoms of women's midlife transition associated with the cessation of periods (a natural stage of life) also called menopause, is now accepted as a deficiency disease. This implies the need of medical intervention, which means adding external hormones, synthetic or bio-identicals, to women's bodies that naturally don't need the same amount as when they were in their reproductive stage (Nature knows best) and by doing so, compromising women's health because they are treating just the symptoms, and not the root cause, and because of the side effects of hormone therapy.

My approach to this important topic is to address it in the most natural way possible, without the use of invasive procedures. Hippocrates' quoted: *"Leave your drugs in the chemist's pot if you can heal the patient with food."* My experience, studies, research, and observation has shaped my philosophy that women at this stage of their lives can keep their health, vitality, and appearance through natural foods and lifestyle choices.

Some of my clients come to me worried about entering or going through menopause not so much for what they hear or because they are experiencing symptoms related to menopause (hot flashes, night sweats, brain fog, mood swings, etc.), but in many cases the major concern they have is about losing youth and

---

15. https://www.health.harvard.edu/womens-health/what-are-bioidentical-hormones

appearance, as many think menopause is the beginning of the end!

Menopause is not a disease neither the end of life, youth, and beauty. All the contrary! We know age is a number. Who set our standards and limitations about age? Is it that our mind has been conditioned by society to believe how we are supposed to look and behave at certain periods in life?

It has always amazed me how two people of the same chronological age could look, think and act so differently; the ones who don't respond to the imposed (or self) limitations of their chronological age are doing things not "appropriate for their age" like starting careers in business, competitive sports, painting, writing, etc., etc. They are curious about life, they don't consider themselves finished products, they discover their true passion and never think about their chronological age, ... or they don't think about age at all. They feel ageless and they look and feel great! In other words, they have this mindset: You are dead when you die, not before!

We also know some younger people who say they feel old and in many cases, they look older than their chronological age...proving that biological and chronological ages can differ quite significantly.

These two quotes by Satchel Paige (a famous baseball player who achieved national stardom as a pitcher at an age when most people have been retired from baseball for many years) will make you think of age in a different way:

- *"How old would you be if you don't know how old you are?"*

> — *"Age is a question of mind over matter. If you don't mind, it doesn't matter"*

In the next Chapter, I will show you how to alleviate the symptoms associated with menopause by **addressing the root cause**; and in the process you can improve your overall health, vitality and appearance. This has been proven over and over, you just need to know how to do it. Throughout this book, you will learn dietary and lifestyle practices to keep your youthful spirit while looking and feeling great the natural way!

Try it out and you will be the best evidence!

V

The Root Cause of Menopause Symptoms. Actions Needed to Restore Health

"The secret of change is to focus all your energy, not to fighting the old, but on building the new" - Socrates

Having this information will save women from a lot of *unnecessary* pain and suffering.

As I mentioned in the first chapter, during my education, I encountered the work of Dr. Daniels[16] who became one of my teachers (I also consider her one of my mentors) and awoke my desire to investigate deeper and write about this topic. In one of her radio shows[17] she discussed the incident that led her to discover that **hormone deficiency has nothing to do with the symptoms of menopause.** Later, during my studies with her, we went over this topic. In her radio show Dr. Daniels explains that she submerged herself in a bathtub with boiled garlic (huge amount of garlic) water which started a severe detox, her liver might have stored well-hidden toxins that were released into the bloodstream and the liver was not filtering fast enough to get all the toxins out of the blood and she began

---

16. Former MD and Harvard Medical School Graduate
17. Is it Menopause, or is it Memorex on Feb.16, 2014 www.Vitality Capsules.com

experiencing unbearable heat and sweat in her body. The immune system in its wisdom pushed the toxins through the skin experiencing something very similar to how her patients described their hot flashes, mood swings, and all the symptoms menopausal women were complaining about when she had her practice. She could not sleep at night, her hot flashes were terrible and the symptoms lasted for several weeks until she brought her body back to balance making adjustments in her diet, cleansing, hydrating, doing enemas, etc. to help the liver cope and the symptoms disappeared. Dr. Daniels helped her menopausal patients applying this approach and they were getting similar results; they didn't need to use external hormones anymore!

This event serves as a perfect analogy of what happens during menopause. The toxins aren't flowing out of the body with the monthly periods (the liver is not prepared for such an unexpected amount of toxins and it can't cope with them fast enough) the body generates extreme heat and pushes out to the skin and dumps the toxins by perspiration which we called hot flashes and night sweats. Toxins also create other symptoms women experience like mood swings, low energy, weight gain, fatigue, etc. The logical thing to do is to give the toxins a better path out of the body, not to add external hormones to an already toxic body complicating things even more.

Dr. Daniels' discovery is indeed revolutionary and very liberating and opens a whole new perspective for women. We know that adding hormones is not the answer because by giving hormones to women, they are also giving women cancer, strokes, heart attacks, ... after all, there is nothing normal about menopausal or post-menopausal women maintaining reproductive hormone levels. Intuitively I knew something was very wrong with that argument. It didn't make any sense to me. Some years ago, in one of my very few visits to a doctor's office (I guess the reason for my visit was to use my health insurance! So I went to an annual physical) the doctor wanted me to start the hormone replacement therapy "if I didn't want to look old" even though I didn't have any symptoms at all. I left his office and I knew I was not going to take that route. I continue living my healthy lifestyle and feeling and looking great, confirming my theory that women can retain their youth, energy, and magnetism through foods and lifestyle practices. No need of hormones, whatsoever! I went hormone-free, with excellent results and this is the same approach I use with my clients who see similar results. Sadly, I also witnessed many of my family members and friends suffering the consequences of the side effects from opting for the conventional treatment.

Following the quote, at the beginning of this chapter, I'm not going to expend more time focusing on the old procedures. We live in times of great changes, therefore I will focus on building the new one, the solution to improve and eliminate all the symptoms attributed to menopause by **addressing the root cause** instead and doing it *the way nature intended*. Fortunately, women have already realized that we have more power over our bodies than we really know and that we can take a more proactive and empowering position. The body will thrive if we provide the right environment: "The best-kept secret of medicine is that the body heals itself if we create the right conditions." In this chapter, women will be equipped with the knowledge and tools to recover and maintain health.

As a result of my extensive research, my education and having gone through menopause myself with no symptoms and no Hormone Replacement Therapy (HRT) or drugs of any kind, I learned to feed my body and my mind to achieve and maintain health, vitality, and beauty. I got this just by having proper nutrition (eating delicious fresh natural foods that have the least toxic effect on my body), supporting the elimination of toxins and adopting specific healthy mind/body lifestyle practices. I knew I could help other women to do the same and this is same approach I use with my clients and they get healthier, happier, and in control of their lives again.

Whether you are approaching the age of peri-menopause, or you are already experiencing some of the symptoms associated with menopause, I have you covered. As we all know, the best medicine is always prevention. The sooner we start, the better! Women who are very conscious of their health have better outcomes. If you are already suffering some of the symptoms, no worries, I will tell you what you need to start doing right now to experience noticeable results in symptom elimination, well-being, and appearance. I will also address and give the solution for other symptoms attributed to the menstruation transition, also called menopause, such as low energy, lack of sleep, weight gain, fogginess, osteoporosis, decreased sexual desire, and more.

We are going to focus on assisting the body by creating the right environment and removing the toxins to create homeostasis to enjoy and to get the most out of every day of our lives. Arthur Schopenhauer stated very accurately: *"Health isn't everything but without it, everything is nothing."*

Cleansing 101[18]: Let's start!

Menopause symptoms are caused by a clogged liver and the toxins floating in the blood causes all these symptoms. **We need to support the liver.**

First and foremost, **start cleansing**. Concentrate on the removal of toxins from the blood. This will replace the missing periods and also **gets rid of hot flashes** and other symptoms. Hot flashes are associated with menopause but many women experience hot flashes before menopause and the reason is the same as in menopause, the body is trying to get rid of chemicals, toxins, and parasites and by doing so women experience a brief fever. It's the immune system trying to remove the toxins or looking for a place to store them and sometimes the immune system will deposit them in places that may cause cancer or other health problems. Hot flashes should not be ignored because they can cause serious issues in the short or the long term[19].

With the following recommendations, you naturally achieve and maintain health. They keep you healthy, energetic and beautiful.

---

18. Basics, Fundamentals
19. Dr. Jennifer Daniels, Online Health Accelerator Program. March17, 2017

The 4 Essentials [20]:

1 Hydrate
2 Increase bowel movements
3 Support the liver
4 Clean up the diet

1. Hydrate

Drink 1-liter of water for every 50 pounds of body weight. Distilled or reverse osmosis water are the favorites.

"It's important that pure water comprise the majority of liquids consumed daily in order to cool the body and cleanse the blood, cells, and organs of toxins and wastes. Water is also essential for maintaining and regulating healthy bowel function and peristalsis." [21]

There are too many chemicals, parasites and industrial waste, such as acid rain and all kinds of things going on in the sky, and a wide variety of pharmaceutical and chemical compounds: hormones, antidepressants, fluoride, chloride, etc. in our water [22]; that is why we need to purify our water before we drink it. Distilled water is empty water it's very cleansing and it creates a detoxifying effect, it's going to flush all the impurities out of the cells, which is great, but also flushes the minerals which are co-factors for your enzymes. Enzymes can't

---

20. Ibid
21. From the book: "Food Energetics" Steve Gagne page 527
22. http://www.nytimes.com/2009/12/17/us/17water.html
https://newrepublic.com/article/115883/drugs-drinking-water-new-epa-study-finds-more-we-knew

work properly if the trace minerals are missing. If you drink distilled water, you need to supplement with a good quality broad spectrum trace (micro) minerals; I like a resin found in Russia called Shilajit.[23]

2. Increase bowel movements

Have 3 bowel movements a day. Because the liver dumps its toxins into the colon you need to be sure the colon is open and working well to move the toxins out of the body.

You can assist your body to get 3 bowel movements by:

Following a 100% organic plant-based diet, rich in real, natural whole foodsthat contain lots of fiber, helps your body to have more bowel movements to eliminate toxins. Do not eat processed foods.

Enemas with salt water. Use one quart warm to touch (about 105 F) distilled water, add I tablespoon of sea salt and mix until dissolved. It's very important to hydrate well before and after the enemas. Lay on your left side. Let the water flow slowly; the procedure should last a minimum of 15 minutes[24].

Enemas: Your best friend. Seriously! As early as 1500 BC, almost all civilizations through history have used enemas to cleanse the body of waste and toxins. Hippocrates used enemas as part of his therapy, it was also a popular practice among the royalty. It was

---

23. https://www.ncbi.nlm.nih.gov/pmc/articles/PMC3296184/
https://www.ncbi.nlm.nih.gov/pubmed/17295385
24. Enemas are safe. It is essential to follow the recommendations on hydration, temperature, amount and kind of water.

included in the Merck Manual of Diagnosis and Therapy until 1972.[25]

Soak in a bathtub of salt water. This will help flush toxins from the cells, therefore, helps eliminate the hot flashes. Put four cups of sea salt in a bathtub with reasonably warm water. Soak for half an hour, preferably every day.

*Bonus: Flushing toxins eliminates mood swings and help you lose weight.

3. Liver support

Coffee enemas The caffeine in coffee dilates the liver's bile ducts, facilitating elimination of toxins trapped in the liver[26]. You can substitute salt enemas for coffee enemas.

Milk thistle, Supports the protection of the liver and promotes its regeneration so the liver can do its job. Milk thistle[27] covers each liver cell and protects it from being killed by the toxins.

For therapeutic and for prevention consume 3 times a week. Use the seeds. The doses: Grind and make a tea. 2 tablespoons, boil in 6 cups of water for 5 minutes, strain. Add more water to make 6 cups and drink one cup a day. Other preparation is to ground them in a smoothie. Or take three capsules two times a day.

B-50 Complex, two capsules a day.

Vitamin C is a powerful antioxidant that protects the liver and relieves pain. Protects against free radical

25. http://www.doctorsreview.com/history/jul05-history/
26. http://suzycohen.com/articles/coffee-enema-benefits-for-you/
27. https://www.ncbi.nlm.nih.gov/pubmed/17133738

damage from normal metabolism, pollutants, and toxins that cause cellular damage[28].

Wholesome real food is always your first option. Vitamin C is found in citrus, fruits, and green leafy vegetables. However, in order to obtain optimum amounts and reach balance, occasional and temporary supplementation is required.

Doses: Ascorbic acid powder. One teaspoon diluted in a quart of water, increase or decrease the amount of vitamin C until stools are loose and then you reduce ½ until the highest dose is when you don't get loose stools. That is your perfect personal dose.

*A minimum supplementation is recommended. Look for supplements that are pure and natural, free of fillers and additives listed as "other ingredients" like dyes (colorants), natural flavors, titanium dioxide, etc. Use supplements only for a period of time, notice how you feel and discontinue when you achieve balance or if you don't feel any difference. Your nutrition should come from eating a healthy diet.

4. Clean up the diet

Start with the right mindset: ***Every time we eat or drink we are either creating health or feeding disease.***

Feed the body properly using 100% organically grown whole foods, whole grains, beans, as well as fresh **local seasonal** vegetables and fruits. Stop the processed foods, white sugar, white flour, white rice… eat healthy real food; junk food does not make you pretty or healthy. To prevent malnutrition, buy mainly

---

28. http://lpi.oregonstate.edu/mic/vitamins/vitamin-C

in the produce section of the grocery store. I highly recommend a plant-based diet with small amounts of quality animal products like eggs, grass-fed meat, etc. if you like them.

Proper nutrition is all about the person's specific needs at certain times and health conditions: sometimes you need to detox; other times you need to build.

Other symptoms attributed to menopause

Lack of sleep, low energy, mood swings, brain fog, osteoporosis, low libido.

Sleep problems

During sleep, the body starts to heal and regenerate and also balances our mood and emotional state[29].

By solving the sleep problem, you also solve brain fog[30] and you will have more energy during the day, not to mention how you feel and look after a good night's sleep![31]

How to have a good night's sleep?

Eat 100% organic foods and especially what grows locally. Pesticides steal melatonin (a hormone that regulates sleep) from the body. This disrupts sleep patters, causing insomnia and a variety of diseases[32].

---

29. https://www.ncbi.nlm.nih.gov/pmc/articles/PMC4651462/
https://www.webmd.com/a-to-z-guides/discomfort-15/better-sleep/healing-power-sleep
30. https://www.health.harvard.edu/press_releases/let-sleep-burn-away-brain-fog
31. https://onlinelibrary.wiley.com/doi/pdf/10.1111/ced.12455
https://www.bmj.com/content/341/bmj.c6614
32. https://pubs.acs.org/doi/abs/10.1021/acs.chemrestox.6b00301
http://www.ajpb.com/news/insecticides-may-lead-to-diabetes-metabolic-disea

- Drink more water, helps flushing toxins out of the body.
- Sleep in a quiet dark room.
- Go to bed at the same time every night and get up at the same time.
- Eat at least 4 hours before going to bed.
- No electronic equipment at least one hour before bed. The blue light that these screens emit interfere with your body's melatonin. Also, use a night light and dim down the bright lights in your environment.
- Practice some breathing exercises to calm the body[33]. Inhale for 4 seconds. Hold breath for 7 seconds. Exhale for 8 seconds.
- Sleep Hygiene principles teach habits you can put in place each day to optimize sleep.[34]

Osteoporosis

Before you run for a pill or a drug please read this:
Osteoporosis is a dietary and lifestyle problem. Bones are a live tissue[35]. What we eat will determine in part how strong our bones will be[36]. Bone tissue has diverse nutritional needs besides calcium; process refined diets depletes the food of important nutrients, vitamins and minerals. Bones are the mineral storehouse of the body. Every time you eat refined, depleted of nutrient "foods,"

---

33. http://www.telegraph.co.uk/science/2016/03/12/simple-4-7-8-breathing-trick-can-induce-sleep-in-60-seconds/
34. http://www.sleepeducation.org/essentials-in-sleep/healthy-sleep-habits
35. https://www.sciencenewsforstudents.org/article/bones-hard-scaffold-influencing-other-tissue.
36. http://www.wellontheweb.net/bone-health-bones-minerals-and-vitamins/

the body has to go to the bones and make a withdrawal of the minerals it requires to help metabolize and digest that refined product.

To avoid or reverse osteoporosis[37]:

- Nutrition: Eat real, clean whole foods. Stop eating junk processed foods, refined grains, flour, sugars, sodas, etc. Excellent foods to keep healthy bones are broths, mineral-rich foods like blackstrap molasses (two tablespoons a day), dark greens vegetables like broccoli, bok choy also called Chinese cabbage, and especially collard greens which is a great vegetable to add minerals to the bones; it is very high in calcium, magnesium and all the minerals to build strong bones.
- Take Bone broth or granulated cow's gelatin. Doses: Gelatin, dissolve one tablespoon of gelatin with a pint of water. Drink once a day. Or add the gelatin to a smoothie. When taking gelatin always drink plenty of water.
- Take Boron in small doses, 1milligram as a capsule once a day. Boron helps promote bone grow.
- Get out in the sun, you need at least 30 minutes of sunlight every day or supplement with vitamin D3 if you live in a location where is no sun for periods or you work indoors. The active form of this vitamin is a hormone that helps bone take up calcium.

---

37. Ibid

- Exercise, avoid a sedentary lifestyle if you want to keep strong bones. Regular physical activity strengthens muscles and bones[38]. Weight-bearing exercises, or any time you put weight or execute pressure on your bones like walking, jumping or any exercise will deposit minerals and make your bones stronger. If your job requires for you to sit all day, stand as frequently as possible, do some jumping jacks, take a 20 to 30 minute walk every day, jump on a trampoline.

Low libido

I learned that a combination of two herbs solves this problem: Milk thistle and Red Raspberry leaf[39].

Dose: Three capsules of *milk thistle* twice a day and 2 *red raspberry* capsules twice a day.

Alternative method: Take two tablespoons of red raspberry loose herb, pour one quart of boiling water over it, steep for five minutes, strain and drink through the day. And take the milk thistle capsules as recommended above.

---

38. https://www.sciencealert.com/here-s-what-exercise-does-to-your-bones
39. Ibid

VI

Healthy Pantry and Refrigerator. Reduce Exposure to Environmental Toxins in your Kitchen

"Let your food be your medicine and let your medicine be your food" – *Hippocrates (the father of modern medicine)*

Despite Hippocrates' words, modern medicine doesn't live by them. We get sick mainly from poor diet and poor lifestyle choices. The current medical system addresses these conditions by using drugs, invasive procedures, and operations that exposes the person to further damage, instead of focusing on promoting prevention through healthy diet and healthy lifestyle practices. Hippocrates clearly stated the connection between what we put in our bodies and what happens to us from the health point of view.

We live in a very unnatural environment. Our food has been polluted by big corporations driven by profits using unhealthy processing methods to create fake chemicalized "food" and by doing so, highly compromising human health.

What Steve Gagne stated in his book "Food Energetics" describes accurately what is the basis of a Healthy Diet, despite our non-optimal environment:

"Naturally grown foods in a semi-natural environment are still superior to those grown in the same environment with all the added toxic ingredients. Therefore, for the best food capable of supporting health, as much as possible and as much as is realistic for you, consume organic and biodynamic foods...Healthy foods do not include foods that have been grown, raised or processed through genetic experimentation, chemicals, preservatives, hormones and other unhealthy measures adopted by corporate agribusiness conglomerates."[40]

The reality is that we are not going to get healthier if we keep putting toxic junk food in our bodies. *To achieve and maintain health we have to take control of how we feed our bodies, becoming conscious about what types of foods we eat and modifying or making adjustments to our diet according to our bio individuality. Recognizing individuality even in a diet is an important concept and understanding that not all foods are good for everybody all the time and specific adjustments in the diet should be implemented in specific circumstances.* By doing this the body starts to balance itself, we feel great and live longer experiencing a high quality of life.

With the above premises in mind, in this chapter you will learn how to build a pantry and a fridge to prepare easy, healthy, delicious meals that help keep you looking young, energetic and happy, yes happy! because the food we eat also has a direct connection with our thoughts, our emotions and our sense of well being.

---

40. From the book: "Food Energetics," Steve Gagne. Pages 530, 531

Make the kitchen the heart of your home to restore and promote health.

I can not emphasize this enough: Fill up your kitchen the best you can, with natural, clean organic unprocessed foods to ensure excellent health and longevity. The purer the diet and with the least external toxins added, the healthier we are. If you are not exactly a good cook and you get overwhelmed by food preparation, not to worry, I will teach you some basics I have discovered: The simpler the preparation method, the tastier the food is with more nutritional value. Use your imagination by adding and mixing your favorite flavors and spices; food preparation can be fun and it's also an art because you can be creative and make your foods tasty, delicious and visually appealing. There is no merit in eating something you don't enjoy with all your senses.

Make sure most of your diet comes from natural foods. Remember to be flexible and follow the 90/10 "rule." Being too rigid and obsessive with food causes much more damage to your health than the "bad food" you want to avoid. In other words, you can enjoy some not so healthy treats as long as you consume mostly healthy, fresh delicious foods on a regular basis and make healthier substitutes for your favorites foods:

> – A cake or a pie cooked from scratch at home with organic ingredients is a lot better than the ones you buy at the store already prepared (you avoid all the chemicals, preservatives, colorants, etc.).

- An ice cream made with just some whole organic frozen fruit is delicious. No added sugar needed. The recipe in chapter 9.
- A packaged organic breakfast cereal is a step forward in the right direction toward health, what makes a huge difference in the number of chemicals and additives compared to the non-organic ones.
- Look at the labels, the fewer ingredients the better. Pass on the ones with a long list of ingredients with chemical names and numbers.
- Buy frozen fruits and vegetables or even better fresh options instead of processed and canned foods.

Benefits of cooking at home:

- The food we cook at home retains the good energy (or bad) infused during preparation. Be aware and impregnate the foods you are preparing with vitamin L (L for love). Food prepared in a perturbed environment is poison to the people who consume it. There is an old saying: "Don't fight with the cook."
- We get to choose and control the hygiene of food and utensils used for preparation.
- We have more control over the quality of our food and how it was produced; the methods and practices used to grow our food are also absorbed by our bodies. I suggest we grow our own food, to buy from reliable

farmers' markets or to buy organically grown food from the supermarket, better than conventional agribusiness foods.

- When we cook for our family and friends we build community, our food will be even more nourishing by sharing and enjoying a good time.
- We save money. Eating at "good" restaurants is expensive and in general not safe. Cheap junk fast food is not a healthy practice.

As a side note, and this is why it's safer to cook at home, I have heard comments from people that have worked at restaurants about "not too good things happening at restaurants' kitchens ... What happens in the front of the restaurant has nothing to do with what's going on in the back, at the kitchen: hygiene issues, poor quality control, not the most desirable energies of the cooks and the people involved with the food preparation... just to mention some of the things going on back there!

Also, do not get intimidated by the price of organic. Remember you are investing in your health and prevention from illness. Prevention is always better: You either pay the farmer now or to the Medical Industry later suffering the consequences of their drugs' side effects, invasive procedures, surgeries, etc. I'm providing here an article from the Cornucopia Institute with great ideas on how to eat organic on a budget[41].

---

41. https://www.cornucopia.org/2015/03/10-ways-to-eat-organic-on-a-budget/

Health Promoting Pantry and Fridge

Start with the right mindset:

"Those who think they have no time for healthy eating… will sooner or later have to find time for illness."
                                                    ~Edward Stanley

A well-stocked pantry and fridge, some basic knowledge about food preparation and a lot of fun and creativity in the kitchen, are your best health insurance.

Staples:

– Cereals, whole grains: Long and short grain brown rice, millet, amaranth, quinoa, barley, oatmeal, buckwheat, etc. Historically people have been eating whole grains for thousands of years[42].
– Dried legumes: black, white and red beans; red and green lentils; garbanzos, mung beans, etc. Legumes have been used traditionally in many regional cuisines for thousands of years[43].
– Sun-dried tomatoes (no additives). Excellent to add to a marinara sauce.
– Good quality extra virgin olive oil or avocado oil.
– Substitute brown rice pasta for wheat pasta.
– Whole tomatoes in a glass jar. Nothing added.
– Blackstrap Molasses.
– Apple Cider Vinegar.
– Vanilla pods or extract.

---

42. http://www.thenibble.com/reviews/main/rice/whole-grains-cereals2.asp
43. http://foodscience.wikispaces.com/Legum http://oklahoma4h.okstate.edu/
aitc/lessons/extras/facts/beans.htmle

- Turbinado sugar. The juice of cane sugar that has been evaporated. Nothing added.
- Spices: Cinnamon, cardamom, cloves, cayenne, cumin, thyme, dill, fenugreek. Spices have both, culinary and medicinal uses.
- Other spices: coriander, rosemary, thyme, sage, turmeric, raw sea salt, black pepper.

If possible, dry, grind and mix your own spices. They usually add additives to them because by law 5% of the ingredients even in the organic version don't need to be listed in the label[44].

Stock your fridge with fresh produce

As stated before, growing your own food is cheaper, you don't need a lot of space to do it, you can save money and it is the freshest most nutritious food you can eat, but if this is not realistic for you, the next best option is a well-researched farmer's market or co-op (cooperative wholesalers): you still get fresh, nutritious food, farm to table style. Get involved and know your local farmers and try to eat local foods that you know have been produced using good practices. Next option is to buy mainly in the produce section of the grocery store and select organically grown vegetables and fruits. When you buy organic you are also avoiding GMO's (Genetically Modified Organisms). You can eat organic even if you are on a budget by using the list from the "Dirty

---

44. http://www.non-gmoreport.com/articles/mar06/non_organic.php
https://www.ams.usda.gov/sites/default/files/media/3 Nonorganic Ingredients -
5% Rule FINAL RGK V2.pdf

Dozen"[45] which tells you what produce has the highest pesticide contamination; therefore buying them organic is the way to go, and it also tells you which ones you don't need to buy organic. This is not a trivial issue, be aware of what you put in your body and in the bodies of the people you care about.

- If you like and choose to consume meat, buy pasture-raised meat, grass finished, hormone-free or organic instead of the commercial, factory-farmed variety. Same for chicken, eggs, butter, etc. Always choose *quality* over quantity. Use animal products as a garnish and eat more vegetables and fruits like in the Mediterranean Diet. Vegetarian diets are a useful strategy for reducing risk of cancer and other diseases[46].

- Raw nuts: almonds, cashews, walnuts, pine nuts etc. and seeds: pumpkin, sunflower, sesame seeds. Keep your nuts and seeds in the refrigerator or in the freezer; buy them raw and store in airtight glass containers to prevent their oils from going rancid; using this method keep them fresh for more than a year in the refrigerator and up to two years in the freezer.[47]

- Dried fruit like prunes, dates, and raisins, etc. (no additives). Keep them in the pantry in a cool place up to three months, or in the fridge or freezer to extend freshness[48]

---

45. http://organic.dev.foerstel.com/the-dirty-dozen
46. https://www.ncbi.nlm.nih.gov/pmc/articles/PMC3048091/
https://nutritionfacts.org/2015/05/05/why-are-cancer-rates-so-low-in-india/
47. http://ucfoodsafety.ucdavis.edu/files/44384.pdf
48. https://www.eatbydate.com/fruits/dried-fruit-shelf-life-expiration-date/

An important note: Properly stored food provides optimum freshness and saves you money:

Do your best to buy only the amount of fresh fruits and vegetables you can consume on a weekly basis (sometimes our eyes are bigger than our stomach) to keep fresh produce from getting bad and wasted. Sometimes imponderables happen that stop you from using your fresh weekly produce, so at the end of the week freeze the ones you didn't consume and used them in green smoothies or to prepare homemade vegetable broths. Also, freeze the scraps of your vegetables to prepare beef and chicken broths. Freeze the bones or carcasses of your beef or chicken.

How to store our food properly is something that someone already figured out, Thank God! Did you know for example that some produce like bananas, avocados, tomatoes, and melons release a gas called ethylene, a ripening agent that accelerates spoilage in the other produce around them that are sensitive to the gas?[49] Or that your root vegetables (like carrots, jams, and beets) keep their nutrients if you store them in a paper bag in the fridge rather than to throw them in the fridge uncovered because they will soften and rot faster? Do you know which produce stays fresher on the countertop? Do you know how to store eggs, dairy, meat, etc.?

Check out these links as a reference for practical storage ideas:

_____

49. https://www.realsimple.com/food-recipes/avoid-premature-spoiling-fruits-vegetables

- How to store fresh produce.[50]
- How to store your dairy products and eggs[51]
- Proper storage of poultry, seafood and meat[52]

There is one topic that needs to be addressed here because of the toxic chemical world we live in nowadays: All the chemicals from our environment we are bombarded with everyday is making us sick. They are called xenotoxins (external toxins) and are found in the air we breath, the water we drink, the chemicals in the food we eat, our cookware and kitchen supplies, in commercial personal care products, air fresheners, EMF (electromagnetic frequencies), pesticides in your food, pest control, computers, etc. to mention a few! Some of these chemicals are not totally under our control, but some are, and those are the ones I want to address here to reduce toxic exposure. This topic alone could easily be another book because this is a crucial issue and it's negatively affecting our health and well-being. I want you to do the best you can to protect yourself and your family from these environmental toxins and endocrine disruptors.[53] The way to do it is by recognizing them and making healthier substitutions.

A healthier kitchen: After all what good does it do to have all these healthy foods if it's going to get

50. https://www.realsimple.com/food-recipes/shopping-storing/more-shopping-storing/how-to-store-vegetables
https://www.rd.com/health/healthy-eating/foods-never-store-together/
51. http://www.wholefoodsmarket.com/about-our-products/food-safety/handling-dairy-products-cheese-and-eggs-safely
52. https://www.realsimple.com/food-recipes/shopping-storing/more-shopping-storing/meat-storage
53. https://www.ncbi.nlm.nih.gov/pmc/articles/PMC2726844/

contaminated with the chemicals released by the pots and pans we cook with?

- Toxic cookware leaches toxic chemicals and heavy metals in our food.
  Try to get titanium cookware or a good quality stainless steel. Ditch non-stick cookware, aluminum, and copper cookware.[54]
- Synthetic chemicals in plastic containers and bottles even the ones that say BPA-Free. BPA is used to give structure to the plastic and it has been replaced by BPS (Bisphenol S) which is of the same family and as harmful as BPA.[55]Yes, very misleading and it's the same reason I don't recommend canned foods especially if it says BPA-Free.[56]They do not tell what replaced the BPA.
- Substitute glass or stainless steel food storage containers for plastic food storage containers. They contain BPA (Bisphenol A) an endocrine disruptor, especially estrogen. Don't use them as containers to store hot or fatty, salty and acid foods[57]. BPA leaches and reaches the food stored in them. Use beeswax-coated cloth instead of plastic bags or cling wrap.
- Make your own kitchen cleaners in seconds using household staples like vinegar, borax and baking soda. Eliminate chemicals as much as possible.

---

54. http://lauratrotta.com/what-is-the-safest-kitchen-cookware-and-bakeware/
https://www.naturalnews.com/036029_cookware_non-stick_chemicals.html
55. https://www.scientificamerican.com/article/bpa-free-plastic-containers-may-be-just-as-hazardous
56. https://www.nrdc.org/stories/9-ways-avoid-hormone-disrupting-chemicals
57. https://www.webmd.com/food-recipes/features/cookware-plastics-shoppers-guide-to-food-safety#1

– You can make your own non-toxic homemade all-purpose cleaner by mixing in a glass spray bottle: 1 cup of white vinegar, ¼ cup of baking soda and 10 drops of lavender oil. Fill up the spray bottle with distilled or purified water. Shake well.
– In chapter 6, I provide an easy recipe to make **Dishwasher, dish soap, and body soap**.

In this chapter, I wanted to concentrate in the kitchen but there is a lot more to say about environmental toxins. I know this is a very important and extensive topic. External toxins could be the cause of many "mysterious" health problems. In chapter 8, I will refer to other common toxins in our environment and how to make healthier substitutions. I think by now you got the message that we have to be aware of and reduce exposure to toxic chemicals produced in a factory that surround us in the modern world if we want to recover and maintain health.

VII

Mind/Body Lifestyle Practices to Bring Alignment to Your life

"The way you think, the way you behave, the way you eat, can influence your life by 30 to 50 years"
- Deepak Chopra

Undoubtedly, there is a mind/body connection. So, in order to achieve health, we need to take the spiritual aspect of life into account, our thoughts, our emotions, our actions to find balance in all areas of our life such us self –love, relationships, career, physical activity... Experience has shown us that we could eat all the healthy food in the world, but if our life is not working or we are dissatisfied in other areas of our life, and we carry unresolved emotional conflicts, our health will be compromised.

In order to experience health, happiness, and enjoy a high quality of life, a **holistic approach is necessary** since we are more than our body. The human body and the mind are intrinsically connected[58]. We can heal the body by modifying or changing our thoughts and emotions and we can also heal the mind by balancing

58. https://www.ncbi.nlm.nih.gov/pmc/articles/PMC1456909/

and paying attention to the body. The body is not a machine where you fix or cut this part or the other…It does not work that way; if the person does not take care of the negative thoughts and emotions that are making the person sick, recovery is not possible.

Hippocrates' famous quote: "Let your food be your medicine and your medicine be your food" refers to the importance of taking care of our physical bodies to provide the right terrain for the body to thrive but Hippocrates also said: *"It's far more important to know what person the disease has than what disease the person has"* pointing out the role our emotions have in the whole picture of health and how our unsolved emotional issues can make us sick.

The food we eat influences our mind and our body. Food is information and dietary intake influences our physical body as well as our psychological well-being[59]. If we eat junk chemicalized food our mind can't have healthy or happy thoughts; the toxic chemicals promote emotional disturbance, moodiness, and aggressive behaviors to name a few… Something completely different occurs when we eat fresh, natural foods; we experience more energy, creativity, clarity, curiosity and a general sense of well-being. There is a connection between food, mood, and behavior.

On the other hand, our emotions, feelings, moods, affect our bodies in two ways: either by contributing to our health and well-being or by the somatization (expressing psychological conflicts through somatic symptoms) of unsolved emotions in our bodies

---

59. https://www.health.harvard.edu/blog/nutritional-psychiatry-your-brain-on-food-201511168626

in the form of aches, pains, and diseases. In an article called "Happiness and Health" in Harvard T.H. Chan School of Public Health on the biology of emotions, the author explains how happiness contributes to health and longevity and how negative emotions and toxic stress harms the body causing "wear and tear," stroke, heart disease, diabetes[60]....

Other studies have shown how in the presence of "positive" emotions (i.e., self-love, happiness) our DNA's coils relax. In the presence of "negative" emotions (jealousy, disappointment, sadness, shyness, distrust, anger, resentment, racism, pessimism, hatred jealousy, etc.) DNA constricts[61].

All diseases are present in our DNA and according to the way we live (how we take care of our body, our thoughts, and our emotions) we either activate diseases or not[62]. We have more control over our health than we really think; this is very empowering if we realize most of our health is really in our hands: By improving our mental habits and behaviors, our body will respond keeping us healthy. So if we want to maintain health, youth and vitality we need to be proactive taking care of our bodies through dietary choices and lifestyle decisions that we make everyday as well as our thoughts and emotions.

Dr. Courtney Griffin, BA at Harvard University and Ph. D. from the University of California and assistant member of the Cardiovascular Biology

---

60. https://www.hsph.harvard.edu/news/magazine/happiness-stress-heart-disease/
61. http://www.encognitive .com/node/1789
62. http://www.bmhegde.com/holistic_lifestyle.htm

Research Program at the Oklahoma Medical Research Foundation, states[63]:

– *"Epigenetic marks are chemical signals that tell the cells which genes should be turned on or shut off."*
– What's more, *"What we are now learning is that the choices we make affect not only our own futures but also those of our children and grandchildren."*
– *"It is kind of freeing to know that we're not locked into predetermined genetic destiny. By making better choices now, you can help yourself, your future kids and their kids." It's up to the individual to make lifestyle changes,* she said.

In previous chapters, I referred to practices to implement (clean food, clean air, clean water and daily elimination of toxins through bowel movements, and other organs, regular exercise, sleep, etc.) to better take care of our physical body by reducing the number of toxins we ingest. In this chapter, we will go over other essential mind/body lifestyle habits (the way we live) that contribute to a healthy and happy life.

My Top Three Essential Mind/Body Tools for Health and Happiness

I want to share these three elements that have contributed to my personal growth and happiness. These are drawn from personal experiences and from the influence of great minds and mentors. I will touch these three essentials briefly -since the subject is complex.

---

63. http://www.33rdsquare.com/2012/02/courtney-griffin-explains-epigenetics.html

I will go into more details later in another book or a seminar but I want to expose you to the following topics:

1. Self-Love and relationships
2. Discover and do what you love to do.
3. "Walk your Talk." Consistency-honesty-integrity

Self-love

When you love yourself you take care of your whole mind/body; making your happiness your priority promotes health and well-being. Emotions have a repercussion in our physiology since emotions alter the immune system. "Positive" emotions strengthen our immune system and keep us in good health; by contrast "negative" emotions suppress our immune system causing illnesses[64].

An Article in *New Science*: "Love yourself to stay healthy" shows how self-esteem has long-term benefits as well as immediate effects on the body. The study at the University of Canterbury in New Zealand shows how changes in self-love produce immediate changes in the physiology.[65]

"In each experiment, higher self-esteem correlated with higher vagal tone. The effect was relatively small, but Martens and his colleagues say this is the first study to show how a change in self-esteem can lead to an immediate

---

64. https://kar.kent.ac.uk/44743/
65. https://www.newscientist.com/article/dn19575-love-yourself-to-stay-healthy/

change in physiology and is an important step towards "filling the gap" between self-esteem and health…

Having high self-esteem doesn't just feel good, it has physical benefits too. It seems that thinking well of ourselves may protect both the heart and immune system."

Why to love oneself first? It is a priority to cultivate self-esteem if one wants to stay happy and healthy as explained above. Besides, like in any other aspect of life, nobody can give of what she/he doesn't have. Perhaps you have been told that it's selfish to love yourself, that you have to put other people first…but, the truth is that the amount of love we have for ourselves is the measurement of the amount of love we can give to others.

Erich Fromm, the famous German humanist, and philosopher in his book *The Art of Loving* explains that a person first needs to love oneself and specify four interdependent elements of love: care of oneself, responsibility to oneself, respecting oneself, and knowing oneself. (e.g. being realistic and honest about one's strengths and weaknesses). In order to be able to love another person truly, one needs first to love oneself in this way. The capacity of self-love is rooted in the same four elements to love others productively[66].

For instance, respect for oneself is honoring one's uniqueness. Be yourself and do not pretend to be like someone else or to be different from someone else. If you have been trapped in the comparison (and competition with others) game you should know that the real true competition is with yourself. You can

---

66. The Art of Loving. P. 26-59

partially get to know yourself by comparing yourself with who you were before and who you are now. Every person has extraordinary capacities, unique skills and talents.

In the world we live in, **herd behavior** is very much encouraged through social and cultural conditioning, subliminal messages, mass media, advertising, education, indoctrination, etc. preventing us from seeing our individuality, our value and true potential. As a result, <u>creating a robotic human</u>, acting like everybody else, doing what society tells them to do, how to look and what to do in order to fit in the matrix to be accepted (using reward and punishment) we become unauthentic people pleasers and approval seekers.

What can we do to express our uniqueness? Is it possible to undo all these learned behaviors that keep us from expressing our true self? We need to determine what of that learned behavior (programming/ conditioning/mass education) is not serving us, questioning everything, unlearning and removing the conditioning, the limiting beliefs, and self-doubts that diminish us and prevent us from seeing our true value and potential and discovering and developing those unique talents.

On the topic of relationships, we express self-love by surrounding ourselves with people: husband/ wife, children, partners in business, family, friends, activities, and situations that contribute to our happiness. When we love ourselves we retain the person(s) and object(s) that contribute to our happiness and remember events and situations that provide us happiness.

I would like to finish with this quote of Kim MacMillen:

"When I love myself enough, I began leaving whatever wasn't healthy. This meant people, jobs, my own beliefs, and habits – anything that kept me small. My judgment called it disloyal. Now I see it as self-loving" –

Discover what you love to do.

Following your passion, doing what you love to do promotes happiness. Because our uniqueness and individuality we all have different talents (which are commonly what one enjoys doing and is good at). By expending most of your time in a job or activity you do not enjoy detracts from your happiness. You could be doing something that you love and in which you would excel; as Erich Fromm quoted: *"Man's main task in life is to give birth to himself, to become what he potentially is. The most important product of his effort is his own personality."*

Discovering what fulfills each of us and by doing so leads to personal realization, one feels authentic and in sync with who one is, expressing one's individuality. We must get out of our comfort zone and expose ourselves to new experiences.

If you haven't discovered what you love to do this exercise can help you:[67]

1. Meditate on the profession or occupation you would do even if you don't get income or profit out of it.

---

67. From the book: "Free-Will the Marvelous Way to Exist" *Voices of Ancestral Wisdom* byAlexandre Sochandamandou.

2. You would never know unless you try! Experimenting and trying without fear, restarting as many times as necessary without changing the purpose.

3. Discovering what you love to do is reflected by the fervor and enthusiasm you carry it out with, the difficulties you overcome, the joy you show when you speak about it and the pride you exhibit by talking about that what you love passionately.

As Johann Wolfgang von Goethe said: *"A really great talent finds its happiness in execution."*

Walk your talk

Mahatma Gandhi quoted: *"Happiness is when what you Think, what you Say and what you Do are in Harmony"*

What Gandhi expresses in this quote, embodies the essential habit to balance the three aspects of our spirit: our thoughts, our emotions, our actions in order to achieve happiness. It requires constant reminding, awareness and continuous practice but its benefits are much greater than the effort.

Make it a habit to be congruent and Walk your Talk. Be the reflection of what you think and say. Make your actions match your words. Teach by example, and by doing so you will develop a strong character, sense of self-respect, congruence, credibility, magnetism and much more.

Last but not least: Three Pathways for Vibrant Health

These three practices are fun and will contribute greatly to your emotional and physical well- being. Personal experience has shown it and many studies are backing this up.

1. Physical Exercise
2. Laughing
3. Learning Breathing

Physical Exercise

Hippocrates referred to physical activity in his famous quote: *If we could give every individual the right amount of nourishment and exercise, not too little and not too much, we would have found the safest way to health."*

Even though we talked about physical activity in a previous chapter as a practice to reverse and prevent osteoporosis, there are a lot more benefits of being active. I have to emphasize this topic here because moving the body and exercising regularly **promotes physical and mental well-being.**

Practicing regularly a physical activity or exercise **that you enjoy doing** like walking, swimming, rebounding, yoga, dancing, jumping jacks, etc. will result in you actually making the time to do it! By all means avoid a sedentary lifestyle because your brain and whole body will thank you.

Regular physical activity not only make us stronger and feel more attractive, but it also improves our thinking, learning, and judgment and also helps us to sleep better and prevents depression[68].

---

68. https://www.cdc.gov/physicalactivity/basics/pa-health/index.htm#ImproveMentalHealth

Keeping an active lifestyle can build strong bones for life, preventing and reversing osteoporosis and other illnesses, cardiovascular disease, diabetes, cancer, hypertension, and premature death![69]

This article in The New York Times (Nov 8, 2007) co-authored by Samuel Wang, Professor of Molecular Biology and Neuroscience at Princeton University, describes the importance of physical activity for the **brain** that gives you enough motivation to start moving:

> *"How might exercise help the brain? In people, fitness training slows the age-related shrinkage of the frontal cortex, which is important for executive function. In rodents, exercise increases the number of capillaries in the brain, which should improve blood flow, and therefore the availability of energy to neurons. Exercise may also help the brain by improving cardiovascular health, preventing heart attacks and strokes that can cause brain damage. Finally, exercise causes the release of growth factors, proteins that increase the number of connections between neurons, and the birth of neurons in the hippocampus, a brain region important for memory. Any of these effects might improve cognitive performance, though it's not known which ones are most important."*[70]

Laughing

Dr. Michael Miller, Director of the Center of Preventive Cardiology at the University of Maryland Medical

---

69. https://www.ncbi.nlm.nih.gov/pmc/articles/PMC1402378/
70. http://www.nytimes.com/2007/11/08/opinion/08aamodt.html?_r=0

Center, says he envisions the time when physicians might recommend 15 to 30 minutes of laughter a day in the same way they recommend at least 30 minutes of exercise.

I don't know if you should have a prescription for laughing but I do know by experience the power that a good laugh has on the mind and the body, and how it enhances our personal and social connections. The added bonus is that besides making us feel good, it's free, and has no negative side effects!

Numerous studies on the psychological and physiological responses to laughter and humor had shown beneficial effects on stress and pain reduction, improving the immune system, enhancing creativity and reducing blood pressure[71].

The explanation why laughter is associated with feelings of wellbeing might be the release of endorphins, also reduces the stress hormones cortisol and epinephrine, and dilates the inner lining of the blood vessels (endothelium) improving circulation. Studies at the University of Maryland Medical center in Baltimore reveals that the act of laughing can protect against heart attacks.[72]

The therapeutic effects of laughter and humor go beyond the physical and psychological well-being. An article of Wayne State University School of Medicine, Detroit, Michigan, Department of Physiology called "Humor, Laughter, Learning, and Health!"[73] refers to numerous scientific studies that have shown that

---

71. http://europepmc.org/abstract/MED/11211708/reload=1;jsessionid=5O3CYj FKTpeNmPJWqQsR.4
72. https://www.sciencedaily.com/releases/2000/11/001116080726.htm
73. http://www.physiology.org/doi/pdf/10.1152/advan.00030.2017

humor and laughter create an environment that promotes learning. *"Appropriate humor and humor that relates to course material, attracts and sustains attention and produces a more relaxed and productive learning environment. Humor also reduces anxiety, enhances participation, and increases motivation."*

So with all those many benefits laughing more should be part of a healthy lifestyle. It doesn't require much effort. Find something funny to read or to watch, bringing humor to a conversation, sharing a joke, making time for fun activities, smiling, and even simulated laughter can be as good as the real thing[74]. Nothing better than a good laugh!

Lord Byron used to say about the benefits of laughter in meetings with his friends, "Always laugh when you can…it is a cheap medicine…."

Learning Breathing

We all have a tool for our disposal that if properly used can help us enhance our physical, mental and spiritual well-being, our breathing! Most of us breathe to stay alive but learning how to breath can add to our health and happiness in many ways … it's easy and it's free!

Breathing techniques as "Pranayama" breathing (deep breathing, or belly breathing as opposed to shallow, chest breathing) has been used by people for thousands of years in India and China as part of ancient wisdom to cultivate physical, mental and spiritual well-being. Now science is confirming what we already knew long time ago... The study is relevant because it shows

---

74. https://bottomlineinc.com/life/emotional-health/even-a-fake-laugh-will-do

how this process works at the cellular and molecular level. By intentionally changing patterns of breathing we can change our emotional states. The article on March 30, 2017, in the Stanford Medicine News Center called: *"Studies show how slow breathing induces tranquility"* researchers at Stanford University found small numbers of nerve cells (neurons) that connect breathing with states of mind. "Mark Krasnow and his colleagues have identified a tiny cluster of neurons that link breathing to relaxation, attention, excitement and anxiety[75]" says Steve Fisch.

When your mood is excited, it is advised to take a deep breath to chill out. In contrast, when your breathing is fast and shallow, tension shows and there is a reduction of oxygen supply to the body cells contributing to fatigue, anxiety, suppressing the immune system …

As part of stress control (stress induces negative emotions like anxiety, anger, frustration but also affects physical health due to cardiovascular disease, obesity, inflammation and immune dysfunction[76]), some practitioners prescribe breathing control techniques like deep breathing "pranayama" (Art & Science of Breathing). Breathing techniques can enhance physical, mental and spiritual well-being. There are several modalities of deep slow breathing but basically consist of focusing on the breath and taking deep full inhalations and slow exhalations.

---

75. https://med.stanford.edu/news/all-news/2017/03/study-discovers-how-slow-breathing-induces-tranquility.htm
76. From the book: "The healing power of the breath" by Richard P. Brown, MD and Patricia L. Gerbarg, MD page 112

Some of the benefits include:concentration and focus, alleviation of anxiety, promotion of emotional balance and keeps you disease-free, lowers heart rate and blood pressure, relaxation of muscles and oxygenation of blood so we think better[77]

Belly breathing is easy to do and very relaxing. Try this basic exercise anytime you need to relax or relieve stress[78]:

1. *Sit or lie flat in a comfortable position.*
2. *Put one hand on your belly just below your ribs and the other hand on your chest.*
3. *Take a deep breath in through your nose, and let your belly push your hand out. Your chest should not move.*
4. *Breathe out through pursed lips as if you were whistling. Feel the hand on your belly go in, and use it to push all the air out.*
5. *Do this breathing technique 3 to 10 times. Take your time with each breath.*

Notice how you feel at the end of the exercise.

An added bonus is that deep breathing is also linked to longevity by keeping telomeres[79] length. During stressful situations, the adrenal glands produce several hormones including adrenaline and cortisol. This response (the fight or flight response) is important because it can save your life. But when it becomes chronic the stress hormones accumulate in the body

77. http://www.ishdhaam.com/pranaay.htm
78. https://www.webmd.com/balance/stress-management/stress-management-breathing-exercises-for-relaxation
79. https://www.ncbi.nlm.nih.gov/pubmedhealth/PMHT0029399/

causing all kind of health problems like cardiovascular disease and poor immune function[80]:

"We investigated the hypothesis that stress impacts health by modulating the rate of cellular aging. Here we provide evidence that psychological stress— both perceived stress and chronicity of stress—is significantly associated with higher oxidative stress, lower telomerase activity, and shorter telomere length, which are known determinants of cell senescence and longevity, in peripheral blood mononuclear cells from healthy premenopausal women. Women with the highest levels of perceived stress have telomeres shorter on average by the equivalent of at least one decade of additional aging compared to low-stress women. These findings have implications for understanding how, at the cellular level, stress may promote earlier onset of age-related diseases…

People who are stressed over long periods tend to look haggard, and it is commonly thought that psychological stress leads to premature aging and the earlier onset of diseases of aging. Numerous studies demonstrate links between chronic stress and indices of poor health, including risk factors for cardiovascular disease and poorer immune systems."

So relax, breath and enjoy a healthy, happy and long life!

---

80. http://www.pnas.org/content/101/49/17312

VIII

Rebuilding our Environment to Create Health

Because this subject is so important for our health, this chapter will be dedicated to bringing awareness about the toxic environment we are living in today and how these toxic synthetic chemicals are destroying our health and our planet. My goal here is to bring attention to this topic so we can make well-informed and wiser choices at the moment of selecting what we allow to enter our homes to protect ourselves, our generations to come, and our planet. Many times people feel sick and they don't make the connections with these exposures and their illness. There is a lot we can do to stop putting external toxins in our bodies and stop polluting our environment by recognizing some of the culprits. I will also provide healthy substitutions (solutions).

Our environment inside our homes is a big problem; we get greater toxic exposure within our house that from outside the house! This is how we introduce hazardous chemicals into our homes:

- **Personal care products** full of chemicals that we put on our bodies everyday: lotions, perfumes, cosmetics, toothpaste, soap, shampoo, deodorant, etc. The skin is a large organ that absorbs chemicals,[81] the same way your intestines absorb what we eat. Therefore, these chemicals are as impactful as our diet because the chemicals in these products are absorbed by the body as if you were eating them. *Do not put anything on your skin that you would not eat.* Minimize or eliminate these chemicals by making your own products with eatable ingredients. For example: Apply a small amount of just plain coconut oil to your armpits, it makes an excellent deodorant. Make your own toothpaste by mixing equal parts of baking soda and salt and add coconut oil to make it as consistent as store-bought toothpaste. For skin soap, use a coconut based soap without synthetic detergents. Look for chlorine-free, fragrance-free, and organic menstrual health products.[82] Instead of sunblock use Carrot Seed Oil that has SPF (Sun Protector Factor) 38- 40. Use common sense and limit your bare skin exposure to when your skin starts getting pink. Wear a hat and cover with clothes to avoid burning. Use oils (jojoba, almond, sesame, olive, coconut or castor) for your face and body instead of creams and lotions.

Even the products labeled as natural or organic usually contain synthetic chemicals and they are not

---

81. https://www.cdc.gov/niosh/topics/skin/
82. http://www.europeanyoungfeminists.eu/2016/07/03/the-dangers-of-menstrual-health-products/

safe. This is what EWG (Environmental Working Group) has to say about organic or natural cosmetics safety:

"Products labeled natural or organic often contain synthetic chemicals, and even truly natural or organic ingredients are not necessarily risk-free. The global market for organic personal care products was valued at more than $7 billion in 2012, capturing the attention of consumers who prefer more natural or plant-based products (Cosmetics Design 2013). Products labeled "organic" or natural can contain petrochemicals, and those certified as organic can contain as little as 10 percent organic ingredients by weight or volume (Certech 2008). FDA tried to establish an official definition for the term "natural," but this initiative was overturned in court (FDA 1998)."[83]

- **Air Fresheners**, are not designed to clean and disinfect the air, they don't eliminate odors, they just mask the odor. They are filled with toxic chemicals: Phthalates[84] which are hormone- disrupting chemicals can cause sterility. Formaldehyde causes cancer of the lungs. Butane is toxic to the brain and nervous system. Acetone is toxic to blood, heart, stomach, liver, kidney. Benzene causes cancer of the ovaries and leukemia. Propane is toxic to the kidneys, liver, cardiovascular system[85]...

---

83. https://www.ewg.org/skindeep/myths-on-cosmetics-safety/#.WkAeniOZOi4
https://globalivf.com/2017/04/17/chemicals-in-cosmetics-can-cause-infertility/
84. https://www.ncbi.nlm.nih.gov/pubmed/21155623
85. https://logisticsconsultinginfo.wordpress.com/2015/04/07/the-dangerous-chemicals-found-in-air-fresheners/

Solutions: enhance ventilation, open windows, use plants to oxygenate your home and clean the air,[86] place some baking soda in a plate and it will pull odor out of the air, use Charcoal-Deodorizer-Fresheners to soak up odors. White vinegar is also excellent for odor elimination and as a disinfectant agent. Use a spray bottle with equal parts vinegar and purified water.

- Also, **clothing** suffers from the same issues described above (synthetic chemical dyes, formaldehyde, heavy metals, flame retardants called brominated, ammonia, etc..)[87]

Solution: Avoid synthetic fibers: Acetate, acrylic, nylon, polyester, rayon. Wear organic cotton, linen hemp, silk, wool, cashmere, mohair, angora, alpaca.

- **Cleaning Supplies:** in the previous chapter we talked about healthier options to replace toxic cleaning supplies:
  Non-toxic homemade all-purpose cleaner: prepare a solution of half white vinegar and half purified water in a glass spray bottle to clean surfaces. Prepare another spray bottle of undiluted vinegar for tougher cleaning. The vinegar smell will dissipate when it dries, but if you don't like the smell of vinegar add 10 drops of lavender, citrus or

https://www.nrdc.org/sites/default/files/airfresheners.pdf
86. https://www.logees.com/cleanair
87. From the book: "Killer Clothes" by Brian Clement, Anna Marie Clement

tea tree essential oil to the mixture. Shake well. Do not use the above combination on wood floors.

Dishwasher, dish soap, and body soap:

*¼ cup coconut base soap cut it in chunks and grated in the blender or a hand grater (when it has been frozen it's easier to grate).

*4 cups of water

*1Tbsp. white vinegar

*10 drops lavender essential oil (optional)

Heat up the two first ingredients over medium heat (do not let the mixture come to a boil) mix with a wire whisk or an immersion blender until soap is melted and the mixture has a homogeneous consistency. Remove from heat; let the mixture cool off and add the rest of the ingredients. Transfer the mixture into a soap dispenser to use as a dish soap or body soap, and keep the rest in a glass bottle for dishwasher use.

Note: It will do a good job but will not produce suds.

– **Use dryer balls** instead of fabric softeners of dryer sheets
– **The chemicals in processed fast food**: aspartame, food preservatives, MSG (monosodium glutamate or additive code 621), colorants, plastics in bottles, and canned foods (BPA a very potent hormone disruptor, acts as estrogen) it is the major

cause of prostate cancer, and other cancers, heart disease, diabetes and obesity[88].

– **Chemicals and preservatives in vaccines** like mercury called Thimerosal which is a mercury-based preservative heavy metal is a neurotoxin that has consequences for our health especially hormone-dependent cancers[89].

– **Wireless devices, EMF** (electromagnetic frequencies) pose health problems like childhood leukemia, Alzheimer's disease, brain fog, decreased levels of melatonin, brain and auditory nerve cancers[90]… electrical devices that produce "dirty electricity" has been associated with cancer, asthma, sleep disturbances, fatigue, skin rashes, allergy symptoms, headaches[91]. Our computers outgas chemicals, PBDEs (Polybrominated Diphenyl ethers)[92] flame retardants when they heat up. Other sources of PBDEs are building materials, synthetic flooring, furnishings containing polyurethane foam, and textiles:

"A number of studies have found PBDEs in house dust as well as indoor air, which is considerably more contaminated with these chemicals than outdoor air. It's

88. https://e360.yale.edu/features/a_warning_by_key_researcher_on_risks_of_bpa_in_our_lives
89. https://www.ncbi.nlm.nih.gov/pmc/articles/PMC4017651/
90. https://www.globalresearch.ca/electromagnetic-fields-emf-extremely-low-frequencies-elf-and-radio-frequencies-rf-what-are-the-health-impacts/5335801
91. https://greenwavefilters.com/dirty-electricity/
92. https://www.atsdr.cdc.gov/phs/phs.asp?id=1449&tid=183

likely that PBDEs migrate out of products like furniture and electronics and wind up in house dust."[93]

PBDE exposure is associated with thyroid disruption, permanent, learning and memory impairment, behavioral changes, hearing deficits, fetal malformation and more[94].

What to do? I'm providing two websites with useful information on how to live naturally in the electromagnetic world we are surrounded by:

https://www.emfanalysis.com/low-emf-internet-connection/

https://www.electricsense.com/3544/wifi-radiation-how-to-protect-yourself/

- Use Ethernet which creates low—EMF, instead of Wi-Fi.
- Disconnect Wi-Fi at night
- If you have a Smart meter on your home, get it replaced with an analog meter or put heavy duty foil, shiny side facing meter on the interior of the wall behind the meter [95] (size 2x2 feet or more) This blocks the signal into the living space.
- Earthing (grounding), walking barefoot outdoors[96]
- If you suffer from insomnia after working on the computer, wear blue blocker glasses.

_____

93. http://saferchemicals.org/get-the-facts/chemicals-of-concern/toxic-flame-retardants-pbdes/
94. https://www.ewg.org/research/mothers-milk/health-risks-pbdes#.WkAabyOZOi4
95. http://www.lessemf.com/faq-shie.html
96. https://www.hindawi.com/journals/jeph/2012/291541/

In the world we live in today it is impossible to avoid all these man-made chemicals someone called "weapons of mass destruction"; to avoid them we will have to live in a bubble! We have created a mess allowing the chemical industry to take over our lives and by doing so producing an ecological and human health disaster in the name of convenience. We know we must stop this snowball in order to inherit a cleaner and safer planet for our children, and grandchildren. It will require for us be informed and change the way we live, being selective of what we buy so industries will be compelled to change the way they manufacture. The knowledge acquired in this chapter is the starting point to protect ourselves and our families. As individuals we can exert great influence; we can be generators of change to protect our more valuable asset: Our health!

IX

How to Get the Best of the Food We Consume. Easy, Delicious, Nutritious Sample Recipes

Mindset for meal preparation

As I previously stated the food we eat take the energies from the person that is cooking the food. If you want your food to taste delicious and be healthy, remember to infuse the secret ingredient: the love ingredient. If you are the cook, make sure to have fun, to be creative and to put all your good vibes and good intentions into the food you cook (forget your worries or distractions). If you don't have the time to cook, ideally have someone that cares for you to prepare your meals.

Food safety:

- Before and after preparing the food wash your hands well with soap and water.
- Change sponges and brushes in the kitchen often (at least once a week) they are microbial incubators and they are breeding grounds for bacteria[97].

---

97. http://www.businessinsider.com/how-often-to-replace-kitchen-sponges-2017-8

Keep a solution of half white vinegar and half purified water in a spray bottle to clean surfaces and soak sponges and brushes. Keep a spray bottle of undiluted vinegar for tougher cleaning[98].

Keep all cutting boards and all utensils clean. Use different cutting boards for raw animal products like meat, poultry, and fish and keep them separate in your grocery bags and refrigerator.

Wash all your fruits and vegetables before preparing them even if you are going to remove the skin.

Cook with clean purified water.

Eating in a relaxed state and in a relaxed environment. Studies have shown how exposure to stress produces an array of alterations of the brain-gut interactions causing all kind of gastrointestinal disorders such as inflammatory bowel disease (IBD), irritable bowel syndrome (IBS), gastro-esophageal reflux (GERD), increase in intestinal permeability, negative effects on intestinal microbiota and more[99]…

Practice a breathing technique (deep, slow breathing) to relax the body before eating to activate the parasympathetic nervous system which controls relaxation, rest and improves digestion[100]. Slow down and breath. The best way for the body to metabolize food is when you are present and relaxed. When you eat in a negative emotional state your metabolism slows down.

Chew. Chewing your foods improves your health helping the digestion and absorption of nutrients from

98. https://davidsuzuki.org/queen-of-green/does-vinegar-kill-germs/
99. https://www.ncbi.nlm.nih.gov/pubmed/22314561
100. https://www.ncbi.nlm.nih.gov/pubmedhealth/PMHT0025459/

your food and reduces your calorie intake because you feel satisfied faster[101].

Tips for cooking:

By now we already realized how important is the food we put in our bodies to recover, maintain, and support the mind/body connection to stay healthy and experience a high quality of life. Unfortunately, because our busy lives, sometimes we don't have the time to prepare our own food and end up grabbing not so healthy foods when we are hungry. This is why planning ahead, a little preparation in the kitchen and learning some basic cooking methods come in handy to support our efforts to stay on track.

In this chapter, I will give you some practical ideas for you to create easy, delicious, nutritious meals every time and encourage you to be your own Master Chef, instead of giving you a long list of recipes, because nowadays thanks to the internet you can find a great deal of them online. Don't be afraid of experimenting (all chefs do) … practice makes perfect!

- Keep at least two sharp knives: A Paring knife and a Chefs knife, will make your cooking experience easier. I'm providing two suggested sources to learn basic and easy techniques on how to use them: https://www.youtube.com/watch?v= ZJy1ajvMU1k

---

101. https://www.webmd.com/diet/obesity/features/crunch-chew-your-way-to-healthier-eating#1

http://www.cookinglight.com/cooking-101/
resources/paring-knife

– When preparing food remember we eat
  with our eyes first; food presentation and
  styling is as important as its flavor....
  therefore, it is important to make our dishes
  appealing to all of our senses. Think about
  the combination of textures, flavors, color.
  Have fun and use your creativity in food
  presentation.

The following recipes are courtesy of my daughter
Juanita Schvartzman who is following my steps with
respect to living a healthy life. These recipes are all easy,
healthy and delicious suggestions not to mention they
are also kid tested!

You can find her at: Yael's Bakery facebook.com

Yael's Bakery (@yaels.bakery) * Photos and videos
Instagram Instagram.com

Chickpea "Cheese"

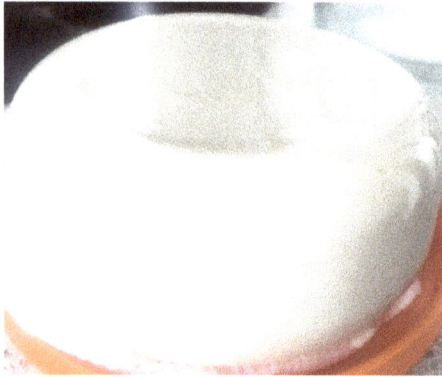

Prep Time: 5 minutes
Cook Time: 10 minutes
Total Time: 15 minutes
Storage: 1 week in the refrigerator

Ingredients:

1 Cup of raw activated chickpeas (approx. ¼ cup soaked overnight)
2 Cups of water
2 Tbsp. Nutritional Yeast
1 Tbsp. Oil of your choice (our favorite coconut, olive, avocado oil)
1 Tbsp. Apple cider vinegar
½ Tsp. garlic powder
1 Tsp. Salt

Instructions:

1. Blend all the ingredients in a high-speed blender for 1-2 minutes until smooth.
2. Place in a pot over medium heat and continually stir as it cooks, you will start seeing it thicken, don't stop until you can see the bottom of the pot.
3. Remove from heat and place in a glass container.
4. Wait until is cold and place in the refrigerator for at least 1 hour.
5. This "cheese" is firm, you can cut it into slices.
6. Enjoy

Macadamia Ricotta

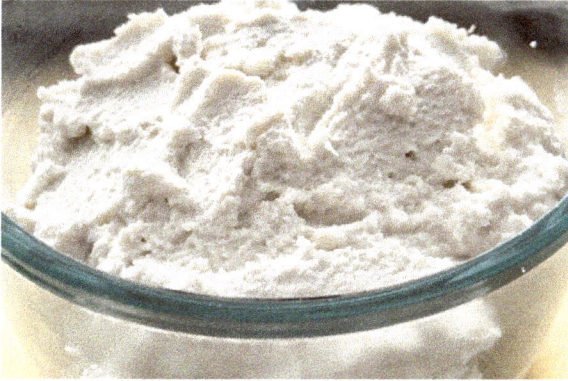

Prep Time: 5 minutes
Cook Time: None
Total Time: 5 minutes
Storage: 1 week in the refrigerator

Ingredients:

1 ½ Cups of macadamia nuts soaked overnight and rinsed.
2 Tbsp. of lemon juice (approx. ½ large lemon)
1 Tbsp. nutritional yeast
1 small garlic clove
½ Tsp. salt
9 Tbsp. water (as needed)

Instructions:

1. Place all the ingredients except the water in a high-speed blender
2. Add 5-6 tablespoons of water and blend on high until it forms a thick paste, scraping down the sides as needed.
3. Add more water, one Tbsp. at a time, until you reach a creamy, ricotta-like consistency.
4. Taste and adjust salt as necessary.
5. Transfer to a glass container and store in the fridge

Melty Mozzarella "Cheese"

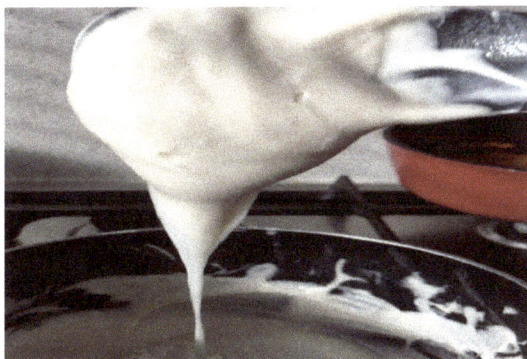

Prep Time: 5 minutes
Cook Time: 5 minutes
Total Time: 10 minutes
Storage: 1 week in the refrigerator

Ingredients:

½ Cup raw cashews soaked overnight
1 Cup water
3 1/2 Tbsp. Tapioca
1 Tbsp. Nutritional yeast
1 Tsp. Apple cider vinegar
½ Tsp. Salt
¼ Tsp. garlic powder

Instructions:

1. Drain and rinse the cashews, add all the ingredients in a high-speed blender and blend until completely smooth.
2. Pour into a saucepan over medium-high heat and continually stir as it cooks, as you stir it will start

forming clumps (don't worry), it will become cheesy gooey. This will take about 5 minutes; continue cooking and stirring for an additional minute.

3. You can Serve hot or
4. Place in a glass container in the fridge.
5. To turn the mozzarella back to its dipping consistency reheat over medium heat while stirring (so it doesn't burn). If it's too thick you can add a Tbsp. of water at a time to achieve the desired consistency

Vegan Cashew Cream

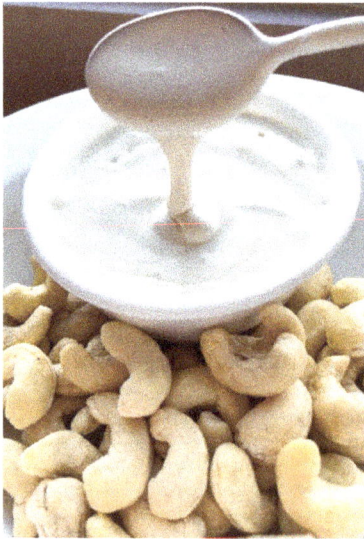

Prep Time: 5 minutes
Cook Time: None
Total Time: 5 minutes
Storage: 1 week in the refrigerator

Ingredients:

1 Cup of whole raw cashews (soaked overnight)
1 ½ Cups of water

Instructions:

1. Place the ingredients in your high-speed blender; I suggest adding ½ cup at a time depending on how thick you want it (you can always add more water but can't take it away)
2. Start blending on low and gradually turn it to high until a very smooth consistency is achieved.

No oil Tahini

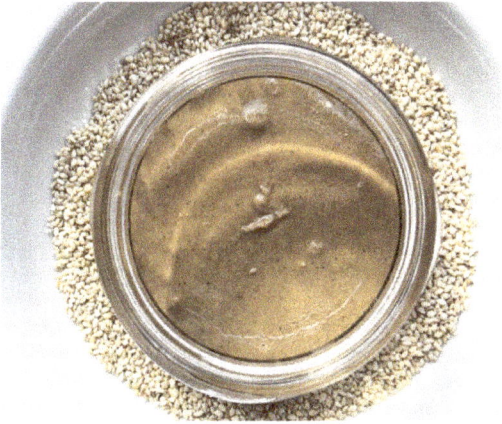

Prep Time: 15 minutes
Cook Time: 5 minutes
Total Time: 20 minutes
Serves: xxx
Storage: 1 month in the refrigerator

Ingredients:

2 Cups of sesame seeds

Instructions:

1. Toast the sesame seeds in a saucepan over medium-low heat.
2. Stir constantly for about 5 minutes until you see the seeds golden and have a nutty aroma.
3. Place in your high-speed blender and blend until a very smooth consistency is achieved.
4. Place the tahini in a glass container and store in the fridge.

Zucchini Carrot burgers

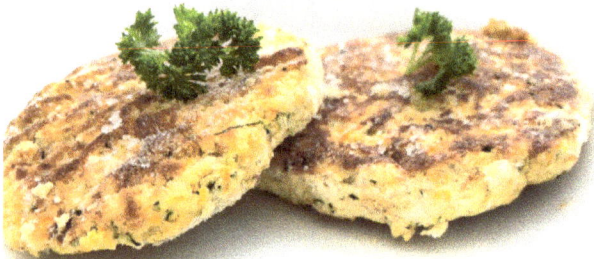

Prep Time: 10 minutes
Cook Time: 5 minutes
Total Time: 15 minutes
Storage: 1 month in the freezer

Ingredients:

1 Cup cooked chickpeas
1 Medium Zucchini, grated
1 Medium carrot, grated
2 eggs
2 Tbsp. Almond flour
2 Tsp. basil, chopped
½ Tsp. garlic powder
½ Tsp. Salt
½ Tsp. Pepper
Olive oil

Instructions:

1. Mash Chickpeas with a fork and set aside.
2. Grate zucchinis and carrots, place in a clean cloth or towel and squeeze as much liquid as possible (don't discard this liquid, is full of vitamins, you can use a base for a soup or smoothie)
3. Stir all the ingredients with the mashed chickpeas until homogeneous
4. Heat olive oil in a large skillet over medium heat.
5. Scoop 2 Tbsp. of the mixture in your hands and press to make a patty.
6. Cook for 2 minutes each side or until golden brown.
7. Enjoy!
8. You can freeze these burgers and just heat them up when you need them.

Cauliflower and Zucchini fritters

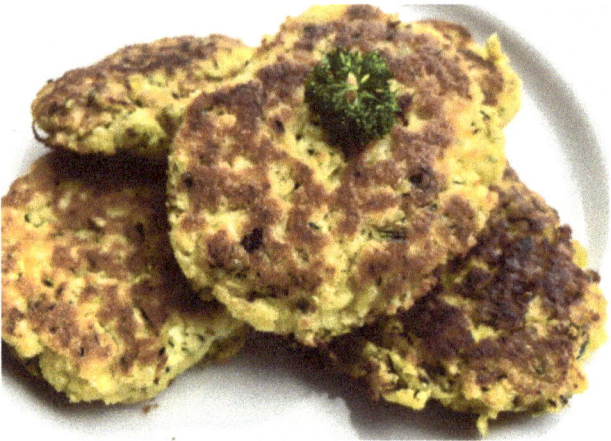

Prep Time: 5 minutes
Cook Time: 8 Minutes
Total Time: 13 minutes
Storage: 1 month in the freezer

Ingredients:

½ Head cauliflower (approx. 3 chopped cups)
2 medium zucchini
¼ Cup almond flour
2 Large eggs
1 Tbsp. Apple cider vinegar
½ Tsp. salt
¼ Tsp. Pepper

Instructions:

1. Grate the zucchini in a food processor.
2. Steam the cauliflower for 5 minutes, until fork tender. Add the cauliflower to the food processor and process until broken down into small chunks.
3. With a clean dishtowel squeeze as much liquid as possible (don't discard this liquid, is full of vitamins, you can use a base for a soup or smoothie).
4. Transfer to a bowl and add the remaining ingredients. Mix thoroughly to combine. Shape into small patties.
5. Heat 1 tablespoon of olive oil in a large skillet and cook over medium heat for 2-3 minutes per side (until golden brown).
6. Enjoy!
7. You can freeze them also and just heat them up when you need them.

Vegan Pão de Queijo (Brazilian "Cheese" bread)

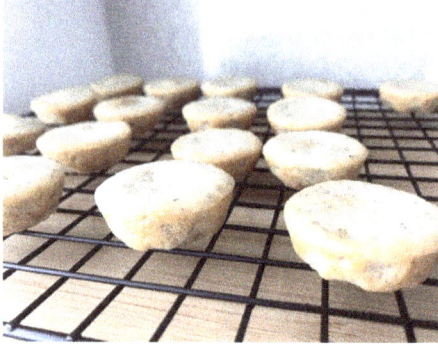

Prep Time: 5 minutes
Cook Time: 20 minutes
Total Time: 25 minutes
Serves: 20
Storage: 1 week in the freezer

Ingredients:

1 Tbsp. golden flaxseed meal
1 ¼ Cup Tapioca
1 Tsp. Salt
1 Tsp. baking powder
½ Cup vegan cheese (I recommend using the Macadamia Ricotta in this recipe)
2/3 Cup of Plant-based milk (I used almond milk)
¼ Cup of good quality oil (I used avocado)

Instructions:

1. Make the flax egg: Mix flaxseed with 3 Tablespoons of water and let rest for 5 minutes.
2. In a food processor or blender place all the ingredients except the oil and blend. Add the oil and the flaxseeds and blend for 30 seconds until smooth.
3. Pour batter into a greased mini muffin tin or a ball-shaped mold (This will resemble better the shape of the original Pão de queijo), but the mini muffin shape won't change the delicious flavor. If any muffin receptacles remain empty, place 1 teaspoon of water on each one.
4. Bake for 18-20 minutes depending on the oven. They should be firm on the outside but puffy. The shell of the Pão de queijo will be very firm when first removed from the oven, but softens to a crisp after cooling.
5. Remove from the tin and let cool down on a rack.
6. Enjoy!
7. You can store this in a glass container up to 5 days (if they last that long) and just heat them up when you need them.

No sugar Banana Bread

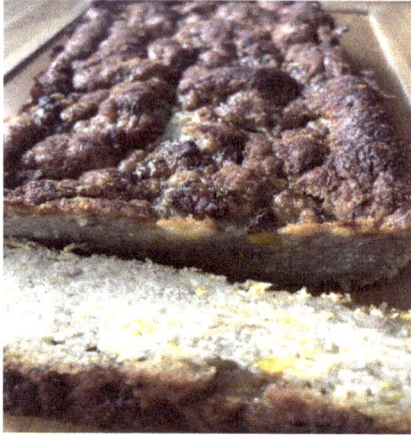

Prep Time: 10 minutes
Cook Time: 45 Minutes
Total Time: 55 Minutes
Serves: approx. 10 Slices (depends on how thick you cut them)
Storage: 3 days at room temperature - 1 week in the refrigerator

Ingredients:

4 bananas
2 Eggs
1 Tsp. vanilla
2 Tbsp. Oil of your choice (coconut, avocado, olive)
1 Tbsp. Apple cider vinegar
1 Cup of almond flour
1/3 Cup oat flour
1 Tsp. baking powder

1/4 Tsp. salt

1 Tsp. Cinnamon

* ½ cup of crushed nuts of your preference (Optional)

Instructions:

1. Place 3 peeled bananas on a baking sheet, and place them in the oven at 350F for 20 min.
2. While the bananas are in the oven, mix the flours with salt and cinnamon.
3. In a separate bowl mix the eggs, vanilla, oil, apple cider vinegar and stir, when is all mixed add the teaspoon of baking powder (you will see it will rise)
4. Take the bananas from the oven and smash them with a fork.
5. Mix the dry ingredients with the wet and the bananas.
6. Pour into a 9x5 pan previously greased and place in the oven for 45 minutes.
7. Let cool and enjoy.

No sugar popsicles

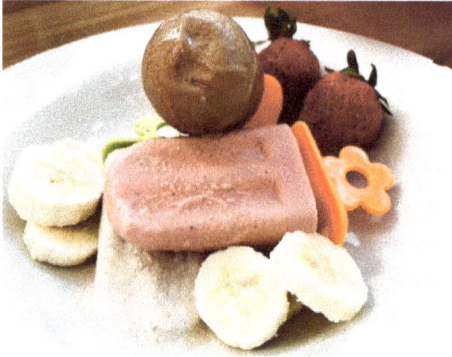

Prep Time: 2 minutes
Cook Time: None
Total Time: 2 Minutes
Serves: 6 popsicles
Storage: 1 month in the freezer

Ingredients:

Base:
½ Cup almond milk (or any kind of vegetable milk)
1 Tsp. vanilla
1 Banana

Variations:

Add to the above mix:
6-7 Strawberries
Blueberries
1 Tsp Chocolate

Instructions:

1. Place all the ingredients in the blender until smooth
2. Put the mixture in the popsicles mold
3. Let freeze until hard and enjoy

Healthy Super Bowls

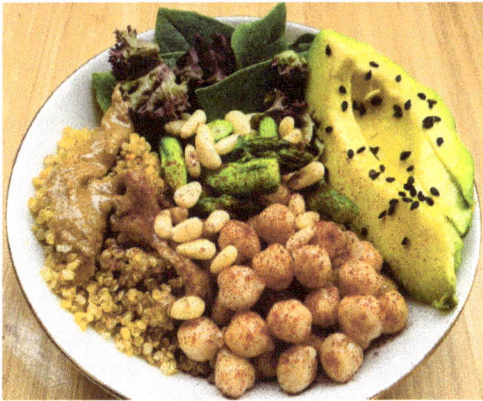

Bowls are very versatile and delicious, here are some ideas. You can make them vegan or you can also add animal protein to replace the vegetable protein:

1. **Choose a Grain** (1 cup of cooked):
- Quinoa
- Brown rice
- Wild Rice
- Millet
- Amaranth
- Barley or other ancient grain

2. **Choose your Greens** (2 cups)
- Kale
- Spinach
- Collard Greens
- Swiss Chard
- Romaine
- Mixed greens
- Arugula
- Any combination of lettuce you like

3. **Choose your Protein** (1 cup of cooked)
- Beans
- Lentils
- Chickpeas
- Green peas
- Poach egg
- Your choice of animal meat thinly sliced or bite size.

4. **Any cooked veggie** (Steamed, roasted, grilled, sautéed)
- Zucchini
- Broccoli (small florets)
- Sweet Potato (diced)
- Carrots
- Peppers
- Squash (diced)
- Cauliflower (small florets)
- Brussels Sprouts
- Asparagus

5. **For fat** (1/4 Cup)
- Avocado
- Any Seeds

6. **Top with dressing** (2Tbs)
- Vegan cashew cream (provided above)
- Tahini Sauce (in a bowl mix: ¼ cup of tahini, 2 cloves of minced garlic, ¼ teaspoon of sea salt. 1 tablespoon maple syrup, ¼ cup of water. Whisk all ingredients to a little runny consistency adding less or more water).
- Homemade salad dressing
- Lemon/Lime juice and olive oil
- Apple cider vinegar and olive oil

Stuffed Mushrooms

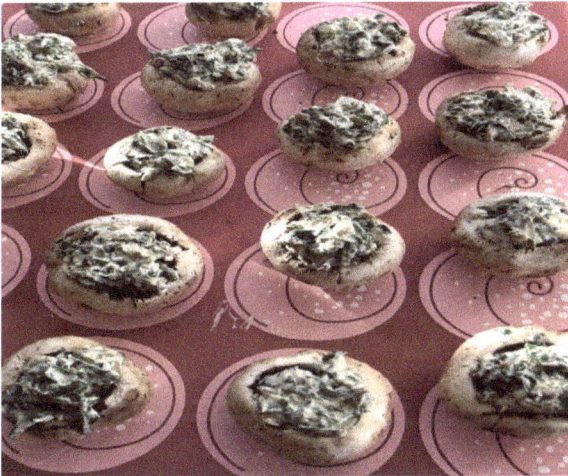

Prep Time: 15 minutes
Cook Time: 15 minutes
Total Time: 30 minutes
Serves: 6

Ingredients:

25-30 medium-sized mushrooms
1 tablespoon olive oil
1 medium onion chopped
4 cups fresh spinach
1 cup of macadamia ricotta
Salt
Pepper
¼ cup almond meal

Instructions:

1. Preheat oven to 375°F/190°C.
2. Remove the stems from the mushrooms. Place the mushroom caps on a baking sheet and mince the stems.
3. Add olive oil in a saucepan and add the chopped onion and minced stems. Stir and cook for 5 minutes.
4. Add the spinach, cook until it wilts, and add the ricotta cheese, salt, and pepper. Stir until the ricotta is melted and everything is well combined
5. Take a spoonful of the spinach mixture and fill each mushroom top.
6. Sprinkle almond meal on top of the stuffed mushrooms.
7. Bake for 12-15 minutes or until golden brown.

Buckwheat tortillas

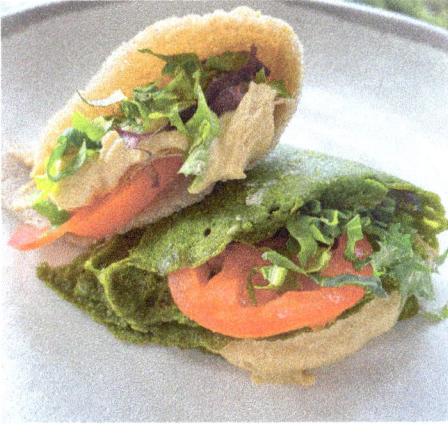

Prep Time: 2 minutes
Cook Time: 5 minutes
Total Time: 7 minutes
Serves: approximately 8
Storage: 1 week in the refrigerator or 3 months in the freezer

Ingredients:

1 Cup Buckwheat groats (soaked overnight)
1 Cup of water
½ Tsp of salt (omit for the sweet version)

Instructions:

1. Wash the buckwheat groats and place them in the blender with the water and salt (if using) and blend everything.

2. Place a pan on medium heat with a little bit of oil of choice, when is hot, add approximately 1/3 cup of the batter until the desired size and thickness you want your tortilla to be (it will look like a crepe).
3. When you see the batter surface drying, carefully flip the tortilla to the other side, let it cook for 1-2 more minutes and take it out of the pan. (The tortilla should be pliable).
4. Do this with all the batter, depending on the size you can get approximately 8 big tortillas.
5. Enjoy.

Variations:
- You can add a cup of spinach for green tortillas or beet or carrot puree to add color and more nutrition.
- You can leave them with no flavor (no salt of sugar) so you can create any recipe that you want, like sweet crepes.

Storage: You can keep them in a glass container in the refrigerator for 4-5 days or put plastic wrap between the tortillas and place them all a zipper bag in the fridge up to 3 months, then you just heat them a few minutes in low heat in the pan before using.

Miso Quinoa Risotto

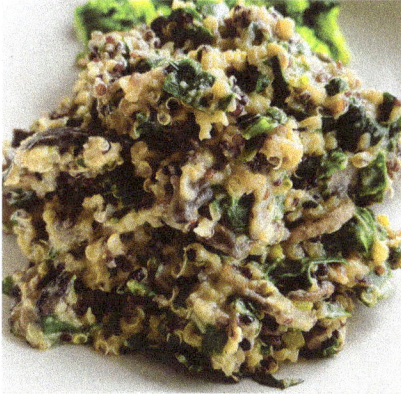

Prep Time: 10 minutes
Cook Time: 15 minutes
Total Time: 25 minutes
Serves: 4
Storage: 5 days in the refrigerator

Ingredients:

2 Cups of cooked quinoa (I like to have cook quinoa in the freezer packed in 1 cup portions).
1 Leek stalk finely chopped
2-3 cups of mushrooms of your choice, cut lengthwise.
1 Tsp miso paste.
2 garlic cloves minced.
1 Cup of non-dairy milk of choice (if using coconut milk, you will have a different but delicious flavor).
1 Cup of chopped spinach.
Olive oil
Salt and pepper to taste.

Instructions:

1. Add olive oil to a heated pan, then add the leeks and stir until transparent, take the stir fry leeks out of the pan and set aside.
2. Add to the pan a little bit more oil and put your mushrooms until golden brown and crispy.
3. Make a hole in the center or the pan and add the miso paste, let it still for about 2 minutes and combine with the mushrooms with a wooden spoon.
4. Add the leeks and the cooked quinoa to the pan and stir in low heat.
5. Slowly start adding the milk and stir until you reach the desired consistency (you may not use the entire cup of milk or maybe need a little more), here you should check for salt and pepper.
6. Add the spinach and let it cook for 2 more minutes and serve hot.

Lemony Zucchini Quinoa

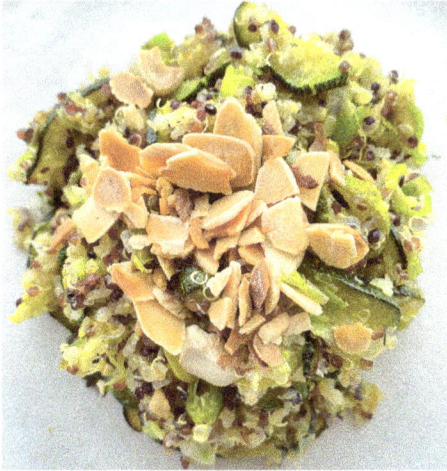

Prep Time: 10 minutes
Cook Time: 15 minutes
Total Time: 25 minutes
Serves: 4
Storage: 1 week in the refrigerator

Ingredients:

2 Cups of cooked quinoa
1 Leek stalk finely chopped
2 medium zucchinis cut lengthwise
Juice of a large lemon
1 tsp lemon zest
1 tsp of dry dill
Salt and pepper to taste
¼ Cup of toasted almonds or pine nuts.

Instructions:

1. Add olive oil to a heated pan, then add the leeks and stir until transparent, take the stir fry leeks out of the pan and set aside.
2. Add to the pan a little bit more oil and put your zucchinis until golden brown and crispy.
3. Now incorporate the cooked leeks and quinoa and stir gently.
4. In a separate bowl mix the lemon juice with the lemon zest and the dill and add to the quinoa, check for salt and pepper and stir everything together.
5. Serve hot with the toasted almonds or pine nuts on top and enjoy.

Blueberry muffins

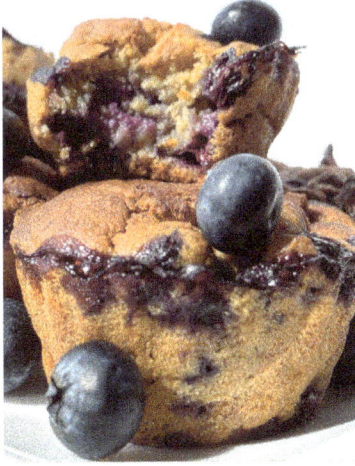

Prep Time: 5 minutes
Cook Time: 30 minutes
Total Time: 35 minutes
Serves: 9
Storage: 1 week in the refrigerator

Ingredients:

1 ½ Cups of oat flour
4 Tbsp Coconut sugar
1 tsp baking powder
1 ripe banana
¾ Cup non-dairy milk of choice
1 tsp vanilla
½ tsp apple cider vinegar
½ cup of blueberries.

Instructions:

1. Preheat the oven at 350F
2. In a bowl mash the banana until very smooth.
3. Add non-dairy milk, vanilla, coconut sugar and apple cider, mix well.
4. Stir in the oat flour, coconut sugar and baking powder and mix.
5. Fold gently the blueberries.
6. Spoon in a muffin pan with paper liners or previously greased
7. Bake for 30 minutes or until a toothpick comes out clean.
8. Let them cool for 10 minutes and enjoy!

Variations:

• You can replace the blueberries and add any other fruit of your choice like strawberries, raspberries, etc.
• You can make chocolate chip muffins by replacing the blueberries for chocolate chips.

Yael's Brownies

These are the most delicious brownies you will ever taste; they are gluten free and vegan. The recipe was developed by Yael Schvartzman, my 7-year-old granddaughter.

Prep Time: 5 minutes
Cook Time: 20 minutes
Total Time: 25 minutes
Serves: 15 brownies
Storage: 4 days in the refrigerator

Ingredients:

1 Cup Almond flour
1/3 Cup of cocoa powder
1/3 Cup coconut sugar
1 Tsp baking powder
3 Tbsp of non-dairy milk of choice
2 Flag seed eggs (1 flax egg= 1 Tbsp of grounded flax seed + 3 Tbsp Water)
2 Tbsp of melted coconut oil
¼ Cup chocolate chips

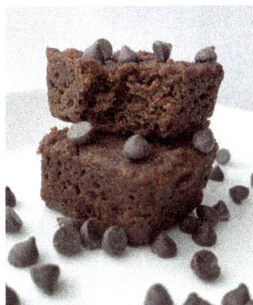

* Optional for decoration: Strawberries or blueberries

Instructions:

1. Preheat the oven to 350F and grease an 8-inch pan.
2. Make your flax seed eggs and set aside for at least 5 minutes.
2. Combine the almond flour, cocoa powder, coconut sugar and baking powder in a bowl.

3. Add non-dairy milk, coconut oil and flax eggs and stir until everything is combined.
4. Add chocolate chips and mix again.
5. Stir in the batter evenly into the mold.
6. Bake for 20 minutes (Brownies will seem underbake but they will firm when they cool down).
7. Take out of the oven and wait until cold to cut.
8. If you want add strawberries or blueberries for decoration and enjoy!

Bon appetit!

Conclusions

It was January the 8th, 2018 a Saturday morning at 8:07 a.m. to be more precise -while I was fixing breakfast at my home in Hawaii and reflecting in the content of my book and the possible conclusions- an emergency alert blurted from my cell phone that made me go and check what was going on. The screen showed: "**Emergency Alert** BALLISTIC MISSILE THREAT INBOUND TO HAWAII. SEEK IMMEDIATE SHELTER. THIS IS NOT A DRILL"

At the moment, I thought, well… living on an island there is not much you can do and there are not many places you can go. Then I thought, if this is the end, I have no regrets, I have lived my life the best I could and if it's over I will face it and stay calm so I can think. This state of mind is something I have learned with years of practicing a lifestyle that supports the mind and the body and provides the balance to remain determined, calmed and in peace (not resigned) even in difficult situations. What would you do if you have ten minutes to live? I continued with my meal preparation…

I also remember I had the song "Moving" from a well known Spanish singer called Macaco playing in the background. The lyrics of the song were precisely what I was looking for and found the inspiration from it to write my conclusions.

"Moving all the people moving, one move for just one dream…" Indeed, more and more people all over the world are getting together to create a collective power of forces to bring a positive vision of our world and the future based on a better relationship with mother nature, living in harmony and synergy with our fellow humans and with all the species we share our planet earth with.

My greatest purpose, my grain of sand, with this book is to provide people with useful tools to make that dream a reality for ourselves but also for our children, grandchildren, … Great advances have been made in the fields of human nutrition and sustainability of our planet. As an example, many oncologists, cardiologists, and scientific studies are showing the association of meat consumption with a higher risk of cancer, diabetes, heart disease and increased mortality, and the substitution of other healthy protein sources with lower mortality risk. Recognizing individuality even in a diet (not all foods are good for everybody all the time and specific adjustments in the diet should be implemented in specific circumstances) there are still changes we can all make like reducing meat consumption to preserve our lives and by doing so we are also preserving the life of our planet.

"Action, reaction, repercussion…" That is exactly the results I found with my research. After all my experience embodied in this book, I realized that its content and practice is useful not only for women in pre-menopause

stage or during or after these changes but also for young or mature men and women who are willing to adopt changes that will lead them to experience physical and emotional well-being reflected in inner peace and strength of character to face all the vicissitudes life presents us. William Shakespeare stated very wisely with his masterly character, Hamlet:

> *"To be or not to be*
> *Whether't is nobler in the mind to suffer*
> *The slings and arrows of outrageous fortune*
> *Or to take arms against a sea of troubles*
> *And by opposing end them..."*

Is the question - to make an analogy - to be or not to be healthy? Being healthy is a decision, there are a lot of *arms* we can use for not getting sick; there are many resources to our disposal to learn from - like this mind/body manual you have in your hands - to live a long life but most importantly, **a high quality life** physically and mentally to leave this planet with dignity. A great motivator, I think...Do the best you can!

In closing, I will say that the greatest changes in the history of humanity have initiated with a few like-minded people; then more and more people join the causes to start producing substantial changes in government's environmental, food and health policies; the latter I consider should be among our most fundamental rights for all people. I feel very honored to be part of this great movement that is changing the world the Natural Way!

It took 38 minutes for a second phone alert to be issued across the state announcing that a Civil Defense employee accidentally pushed the alert button! That means dear readers we all have the opportunity to live the best life each of us can every moment while we are still alive…we never know when life is going to end, and now it is the moment to build a happier, **safer**, and less toxic World for all.

References

Brown, Richard P. MD and Gerbarg, Patricia L. MD (2012) *The healing power of breath.* Shambhala Publications, Inc. Boston, Massachusetts.

Bieler, Henry G. MD (1965) Food Is Your Best Medicine. The Random House Publishing Group.

Casper, M J (2003) *Synthetic Planet. Chemical politics and hazardous of modern life.* Routledge. Great Britain.

Clement, A.M. and Clement B. *Killer Clothes.* (2011) Hippocrates Publications. Summertown, TN.

Gagne, Steve (2008) *Food Energetics.* Healing Arts Press. Rochester, Vermont.

Hegde, B M. (2017) *What Doctors Don't get to Study in Medical School.* Paras Medical Publisher. Hyderabad, India.

Jensen, B. *Tissue Cleansing Through Bowel Management.* (1981) Healthy Living Publications. Summertown, TN.

Singer, Ross Sydney (1995, 2002, 2006) Dressed to Kill. Avery Publishing Group

Watkins, Elizabeth E. (2010) *The Estrogen Elixir.* The Hopkins University Press. Baltimore, Maryland.

.

www.ingramcontent.com/pod-product-compliance
Lightning Source LLC
Chambersburg PA
CBHW050842270326
41930CB00019B/3444